PRAISE FOR
YOUR EXCEPTIONAL LIFE

"I have had the opportunity to be interviewed by Marcus a number of times as well as have him in attendance at one of my signature seminar programs, The Breakthrough Experience. His dedication to self-mastery and his work uncovering the lives of the men and women outlined in his new book *Your Exceptional Life* is exactly that, exceptional. It is a masterpiece for creating a magnificent life. If you would love to master your life as *The Exceptionals* have demonstrated and desire longevity, inspiration and an extraordinary fulfilled life, this book is for you."
Dr John Demartini – International bestselling author of *The Values Factor*

"This book is going to change lives!"
Laura Barry – Teacher and parent

"You can tell Marcus has dug incredibly deep to bring this book to the world. *The Exceptionals* are inspiring, the memoirs are so vulnerable and authentic, and the pathway laid out is well researched, practical and achievable."

Kate Raines – Psychotherapist and personal trainer

"*Your Exceptional Life* illustrates what it means to live an extraordinary life, by beautifully bringing to life the stories of some incredibly inspiring people. But inspiration isn't enough anymore. Marcus distils this inspiration into some simple but practical easy steps. It's like having a personal concierge for every aspect of your life so that you too can make the rest of your life the best of your life."

Peter Lennon – Father to five, coach and host of *The U Matter Project*

"Only special people can see what Marcus sees. The way he educates from his interpretation of the data is genius-like. The stories he tells and the adventure he takes you on in this book will have you reading and rereading this incredible piece of work over and over, so that you can take positive strides towards becoming the most exceptional version of yourself."

Damian Kristof – Naturopath, nutritionist, chiropractor and co-host of *100 Not Out*

"Marcus Pearce personifies exceptional. In his book he highlights people who have lived exceptional lives. He also gives you the blueprint to be exceptional. I know Marcus. He is happy, healthy, wealthy, witty, enthusiastic and charming. What better narrator and teacher is there than one that lives an exceptional life. Reading *Your Exceptional Life* is life-changing."

Cyndi O'Meara – Founder and creative director of Changing Habits and The Nutrition Academy

"The delivery of Marcus's vast wisdom is delightful, entertaining and always inspiring."

Bronnie Ware – International bestselling author of *The Top Five Regrets of the Dying*

"'Extremely good or impressive in a way that is unusual' is the dictionary meaning of 'exceptional' and Marcus Pearce has encapsulated the exceptional meaning wholeheartedly in this phenomenal new book. Far from being the predictable monotone of the thousands of self-help books available, Marcus has managed to use compelling real-life stories and principles to help the reader feel truly inspired and able to implement change with ease. His unique delivery masterfully propels you to want to make the rest of your life the best of your life. It is the number one book every exceptional human will be devouring."

Kim Morrison – International bestselling author of *The Art Of Self Love* **and founder of Twenty8 Essentials**

YOUR
EXCEPTIONAL
LIFE

MAKE THE REST OF YOUR LIFE
THE BEST OF YOUR LIFE

YOUR EXCEPTIONAL LIFE

MAKE THE REST OF YOUR LIFE
THE BEST OF YOUR LIFE

MARCUS PEARCE

First published in 2021 by Dean Publishing
PO Box 119
Mt. Macedon, Victoria, 3441
Australia
deanpublishing.com

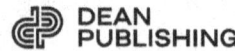

Copyright © Marcus Pearce

All rights reserved. No part of this publication may be reproduced, stored in a retrieval system or transmitted in any way or by any means, electronic, mechanical, photocopying, recording or otherwise, without the prior written permission of the author.

Cataloguing-in-Publication Data
National Library of Australia
Title: Your Exceptional Life — Make The Rest Of Your Life The Best Of Your Life
Edition: 1st edn
ISBN: 978-1-925452-32-7
Category: Self-Help/Personal Growth/General

Cover Design: Jazmine Morales
Cover Image: Sarah Hill

The information provided in this book is designed to provide helpful information on the subjects discussed. This book is not meant to be used, nor should it be used, to diagnose or treat any physical, emotional or psychological medical condition. For diagnosis or treatment of any medical problem, consult your own physician. The publisher and author are not responsible for any specific health or psychological needs that may require medical supervision and are not liable for any damages or negative consequences from any treatment, action, application or preparation, to any person reading or following the information in this book. References are provided for informational purposes only and do not constitute endorsement of any websites or other sources. Neither the publisher nor the individual author(s) shall be liable for any physical, psychological, emotional, financial, or commercial damages, including, but not limited to, special, incidental, consequential or other damages. Our views and rights are the same: You are responsible for your own choices, actions, and results.

*For Maya, Darby,
Tommy and Spencer*

There is more to the story in the INTERACTIVE book.

See exclusive behind-the-scenes videos, audios and photos.

DOWNLOAD it for free at deanpublishing.com/exceptional

CONTENTS

Foreword   iii

Preface   vii

Introduction   xiii

PART ONE
YOUR EXCEPTIONAL LONGEVITY

LIFE PURPOSE   3

MOVEMENT   43

SOCIAL LIFE   65

PART TWO
YOUR EXCEPTIONAL QUALITY OF LIFE

NUTRITION   89

FAMILY   117

GROWTH   169

WEALTH   185

PART THREE
YOUR EXCEPTIONAL SPIRIT

SPIRIT   217

▲ ▲ ▲

Afterword	261
Acknowledgements	263
Bibliography	267
Cast of The *Exceptionals*	273
Create Your Exceptional Life	275
About The Author	279
Endnotes	281
Permissions	295

FOREWORD

I remember it like it was yesterday. The year was 2008, and I had just arrived back in Melbourne from five years in New Zealand, where I had been studying and hosting a healthy weight loss TV show called *Downsize Me!* I had launched a new breakfast brand and was travelling the country to present a seminar called *The Power of Food*. I was approached by Marcus and his wife, Sarah, to give this talk in regional Victoria. Unbeknownst to me at the time, this connection would become one of the most rewarding friendships of my entire life.

Marcus, arguably the most enthusiastic person I had ever come across, was set to send me down the rabbit hole of health and wellbeing at a time when I thought I had learned everything I needed to know. Having spent the best part of a decade studying nutrition, naturopathy and chiropractic, I felt as if I was bursting with knowledge. But boy oh boy, was I about to be shown how much I still had to learn!

In 2013 and on the eve of my 40th birthday, Marcus suggested that we could do a podcast together on ageing well. Marcus, an already keen longevity enthusiast and researcher, had a genuine fascination with living your best life. In fact, his modus operandi had become living an *exceptional* life. I was becoming more and more daunted about the prospect of turning 40 and 'over the hill'. I was scared that my best years were behind me and felt myself succumbing to some 'stinking thinking' that the future would not be as good as the past.

In preparation for our podcast, Marcus sent me an ABC documentary *The 100+ Club* and a variety of book summaries, news articles and more that all began to subtly inform me that I was miles away from getting or even being old. I was hooked and so began the *100 Not Out* podcast, our journey and exploration into what we reverently refer to as mastering the art of ageing well.

In the first 10 or so episodes, it became crystal clear that my understanding of longevity, nutrition, lifestyle, family and values was about to be turned upside-down. Australia's oldest man, Dexter Kruger, told us that he enjoyed coffee and cake twice a day with friends before having another coffee at midnight! Centenarian Ruth Frith was winning World Masters Games gold medals and told us her exercise routine was more important than her diet, especially because she did not eat vegetables! Dr Walter Bortz, author of *The Roadmap to 100*, had also proclaimed that movement was more influential on graceful ageing than nutrition.

Time and again, the life experiences of our guests were shattering my long held beliefs about ageing. The tipping point came in 2016 when Marcus and I hosted our first 10-day Longevity Experience on the Greek island of Ikaria – colloquially known as 'the island where people forget to die'. After immersing myself in the lifestyle of the Ikarians, I decided to rip up my own book manuscript. I had come to realise that almost everything I was taught in spending a decade at college and at seminars was not necessarily wrong – but not necessarily right either. There were more pieces in the puzzle of living a healthy and long life than what budding health professionals were being taught at university.

What you'll discover in this book is the complete set of puzzle pieces. Marcus calls this the Exceptional Life Blueprint, and *The Exceptionals* featured in this book are the roadmap to help you live your own magnificent life.

FOREWORD

You are about to go on a journey of discovery as to how you can transform and improve your life to be exponentially better than what it is right now – even if you absolutely love your life. You won't find complex solutions that are impossible to achieve; instead the book you hold in your hands will return you to a simplicity and ease many of us believe is no longer possible. I promise you, having transformed my own life and belief system and witnessed it in thousands of others, living an exceptional life is yours for the taking.

This book is your opportunity to elevate the areas of your life from what you consider to be mediocre or sub-par to exceptional. I am fortunate in my life to have been able to learn much of this with and from Marcus. However, in reading this masterpiece, I also realise that the life perspective Marcus has is one not many people do. Only special people can see what he sees. How Marcus educates from his interpretation of the data is genius-like. The stories he tells and the adventure he takes you on in this book will have you reading and rereading this incredible piece of work, so that you can take positive strides towards becoming the most exceptional version of yourself.

Take care,

Dr Damian Kristof
Chiropractor – Naturopath – Nutritionist
damiankristof.com

PREFACE

From Red Bull and Cigarettes to Ginger Tea

Like many Australian children in the 1980s, I grew up on a daily diet of Rice Bubbles and two pieces of Vegemite toast for breakfast, two Mint Slices for morning tea, a stale white bread margarine-lathered peanut butter sandwich for lunch, Barbecue Shapes for afternoon tea, pasta for dinner, and ice cream with Milo for dessert. I have no memories of drinking water as a child; instead I was constantly sipping on super sweet lemon cordial and soft drinks.

Ask 100 people born in the 1980s in Australia and I'm sure you'll find my childhood diet, whilst definitely unhealthy, was not uncommon for an Australian child growing up at that time.

My parents split up when I was 10, which was naturally heartbreaking. In hindsight it was the best decision they ever made. Ever since I can remember I knew I wanted to be a sports journalist. I studied journalism at university, worked in radio for five years before landing a plum job as Associate Producer of *The AFL Footy Show*, at the time the number one live television show in Australia. Whilst many closest to me may have felt this was the next big step of a lifetime media career, I was about to transform in a completely different way.

I had fallen in love with an incredible woman who was different to me in almost every way you can imagine. Sarah (now my beautiful wife) was a health professional with a high value on eating well, work-life balance, and an overall healthy lifestyle. I on the other hand was a work-hard, play-hard journalist who loved smoking, binge drinking and had an 'anything goes' laissez-faire relationship with food.

And whilst the sparks of romance were flying in all directions, my decade-long smoking habit and 'everything in generous moderation' health philosophy was not exactly advancing our relationship. One particularly distasteful experience took place early each Friday morning. *The Footy Show* went to air every Thursday night, and I'd return home in the early hours of the morning smelling like cigarettes and beer. Too tired to shower, I'd crawl straight into bed next to Sarah. My girlfriend of a few months would be startled awake by the disgusting stench that had entered her peaceful slumber. It was not a good look! After a number of agitated Friday morning conversations, I decided to do something about it.

My love of statistics would help me quit smoking. My three-cigarette per day habit had to sound and feel a whole lot worse than that. I calculated that three cigarettes per day was in fact over 1000 per year, and more than 10,000 per decade. If I was going to enjoy a lifetime relationship with Sarah and have children with her (and be a great example to them), then smoking just simply wasn't going to work. Without intending to oversimplify it, this understanding was all I needed to quit. I had to make smoking inconsistent with my identity.

My personal changes didn't stop with smoking. I also went on a 30-day meat-free challenge, and as a result my nickname at work went from 'MP' or 'Pearcey' to 'Mung Bean'! I swapped my morning tea Red Bull and cigarette for a freshly-grated ginger tea and cashew nuts, and the chicken schnitzel burger I once chowed down for lunch was now a chickpea curry and rice at the local Indian vegetarian café. By 2005 I was a non-smoking, five kilograms lighter vegetarian-soon-to-become vegan. I felt unstoppable. And at 24 years of age, I felt I'd reached enlightenment sooner than I expected. The secrets to longevity and an exceptional life were as simple as removing animal products and cigarettes (or at least that's what I thought).

In 2006 I said goodbye to the media, travelled the world with Sarah for 18 months, returned home to live by the sea in country Victoria, founded a wellness centre, got married, and started a family.

Searching for the fountain of youth

By 2010 I was a raging vegan and truly believed that a vegan lifestyle (no meat, dairy, animal products of any kind – not even honey) was the official fountain of youth and key ingredient to a great long life. On top of that, I'd given up alcohol four years earlier and believed all alcohol was bad for you.

And then one night my world turned upside down. As a voracious reader and someone continually looking to have my views reaffirmed, I began reading a book called *Healthy at 100* by renowned vegan John Robbins (b. 1947). I expected this book to reaffirm to me that being a vegan was not only the best decision one could make in life, but also for longevity.

My beliefs were about to be slapped in the face.

Robbins grew up the heir to the throne of Baskin Robbins ice cream – a multi-billion dollar global ice cream franchise you have most likely enjoyed at least once in your life. Robbins grew up eating ice cream for breakfast, lunch and dinner, spending his summer holidays playing in his ice cream shaped swimming pool, and being groomed to take over the family business.

Robbins didn't like what he was seeing though. His uncle, and co-founder, Burt Baskin, died of a heart attack at 54, and his father, Irv Robbins had diabetes, high blood pressure and high cholesterol. After renouncing himself from the family business, John and his wife, Deo, left for Canada, where they lived in a small hut, sprinkled cabbage seeds in the backyard, taught meditation and yoga for gold coin donations, and lived on their crops. In short, Robbins's life took a 180-degree turn, culminating in a career as an author of many books including *Healthy at 100*, *Diet For A New America* and *Food Revolution*.

I was no further in to the book than page two of the introduction when my own life took a sharp turn. Robbins was referring to a study completed by the Yale School of Public Health. The results of it changed my life completely.

In the study, more than 600 men and women were asked multiple times over the course of 20 years whether they agreed with statements including: 'As you age you become less useful', 'As you age you become more of a liability', and 'As you age your best years are behind you'.[1]

What the study found was that the people who agreed with these statements had a disempowered view of ageing, dying on average 7.5 years earlier than those who disagreed. What fascinated me and sent shivers down my spine was that they didn't measure their exercise, genes, economic status, family life, careers or environmental factors.[2]

All they measured was a *belief*.

Most glaring of all for me, was that they didn't measure their diets. This hit me between the eyes. All it took was two pages from a book written by a legend of the vegan world to show me the fountain of youth did not live in our diet. The best thing about being a journalist is that I didn't take this personally. Instead of judging myself, I became intensely curious. The next day, I went to work at our wellness centre and paid particular attention to everyone coming in. I was on a mission to see if this belief of a disempowered future was as widespread as Robbins proclaimed.

One after another, all I heard from Sarah's patients was "I'm too old to do this" and "I'm too old to do that". I was shocked by how disempowered people had become all because of a number – and some of these people were only in their twenties and thirties.

I was so rocked by my findings that I decided to put my journalist hat back on and go on the hunt for people who were ageing well. I didn't want my research to start and end at our wellness centre or with the remote cultures Robbins had featured in his book. I wanted to find more relatable people living relatable lives.

"How you age is negotiable."
– **Dr Walter Bortz**

A blueprint for life reveals itself

Research is a wonderful thing when you're learning information that inspires you. Minute by minute, day by day, I felt my beliefs changing about what it took to live an exceptional life. I was coming across human beings that were living simply remarkable lives, and whilst they were impacting me greatly, I just knew I had to share their stories with the world.

By 2012, podcasts had become a great way to share a message, and so without more than a moment's thought, I called my good friend Dr Damian Kristof, a health professional and media identity in Melbourne who was 39-about-to-turn-40 and not looking forward to it. I pitched the idea of co-hosting a podcast on longevity. He said yes, and we were off. The *100 Not Out* podcast was born.

As a vegan (and despite my epiphany), I still believed that we would find a vegan diet to be a strong precursor to both quantity and quality of life. Damian, a strict omnivore (meat, grains, vegetables, dairy, nuts and seeds), held the view that we would find that this style of eating was the most important factor in living a long life.

We conducted our first 12 interviews in less than two days, and it was clear that our respective biases were anecdotally being smashed to pieces. Ruth Frith, who won World Masters Athletics gold medals at 101, didn't eat vegetables. Fitness fanatic and Australian football legend, Tommy Hafey, ate ice cream every day. Octogenarian Mimi Kirk meanwhile had moved from a vegetarian diet to vegan diet in order to improve her arthritis, and thrived.

With every passing guest a blueprint for living a great, long life was revealing itself. Diet was *not* the number one ingredient. In fact, founders and formulators of the internationally acclaimed Atkins, South Beach and Pritikin diet all died at 72 or younger. And if our guests were anything to go by, movement in any form was far more important than society, medicine and governments had been telling us.

But it wasn't as simple as working out the importance of diet versus exercise. What about career choice, relationships, wealth and spirituality? Where did they fit into the hierarchy of living a great life? What impact did stress and trauma have on longevity? I asked myself these questions for years, interviewing dozens of living legends in search of the answers. Countless nights were spent pondering the research, and eventually it struck me that no matter your genes, upbringing, race, religion, culture, financial status or diet, there was a pattern – a blueprint – for being truly exceptional in each area of life and not just one. It was at that moment the Exceptional Life Blueprint was born.

Before we dive deep into this blueprint, allow me to introduce you to the people who inspired it – people I like to call *The Exceptionals*.

INTRODUCTION

Meet *The Exceptionals*

The happiest man you'll ever meet is centenarian Holocaust survivor, Eddie Jaku OAM (b. 1920). Every family member, except his sister, was murdered by the Nazis. His parents, siblings, grandparents, aunties, uncles and cousins all perished. Despite these atrocities, Jaku today is a loving husband, father, grandfather and great-grandfather. He is *Exceptional* in every sense of the word.

Florence Nightingale (1820–1910) was born at a time when life expectancy was 41 years of age and women were expected to be a wife and mother. Nightingale felt called to devote her life to the service of others, and despite the intense opposition from her family, Nightingale went on to become the founder of modern nursing and is renowned for professionalising nursing roles for women. 'The lady with the lamp', as Nightingale was known, lived to the age of 90.

Dexter Kruger (b. 1910) started writing at 86 years young, and retired from farming at 95. He enjoys coffee and cake with friends twice per day and drinks a coffee at midnight to help him sleep. He breaks most, if not all of the well-held nutrition guidelines. Despite being blind, Kruger is a prolific author and at the time of writing he is not only Australia's oldest man, but the world's oldest active author.

Sister Madonna Buder (b. 1930) started running at 48. At 82, Buder became the oldest woman to ever finish an Ironman Triathlon (i.e. a 3.8 km swim, 180km bike ride and 42.2km run) when she crossed the finish line under the 17-hour cutoff at the 2012 Ironman Canada. Buder, known as the 'Iron Nun', has completed over 300 triathlons including 45 Ironman distances.

The small Greek island of Ikaria is known as 'the island where people forget to die'. Ikarians drink generous amounts of coffee and wine, love their bread and many of them smoke. Ikarians experience 80% less dementia, 50% less heart disease and 20% less cancer than the western world.[3] Ikaria is one of only five official 'Blue Zones' on the planet – locations where people live longer, healthier lives than the rest of the world.

These people are just a few of *The Exceptionals*, the small percentage of humanity who make the rest of their life the best of their life, no matter what has happened in the past. This book is your invitation to join them. To be an *Exceptional* you don't need extreme wealth, fame, beauty or the best genes. Instead, membership to this exclusive club requires that you question the many conventional and limiting beliefs thrust upon you by a unique yet overwhelming selection of family, friends, colleagues, media and society as a whole.

The problem for most of us however, is our belief that we are too busy to be exceptional.

Busy and overwhelmed on repeat

If you're like most people I've worked with over the years, you have at certain times in life become so busy being busy that the feeling of overwhelm feels almost normal. On top of that, it feels repetitive like the thump thump of the treadmill or pitter-patter of the hamster wheel.

Just like Bill Murray in the iconic film *Groundhog Day*, you may feel like the daily repeat cycle is here to stay. Whether it is the daily grind of school, raising children, carving out a career, a marriage, a social life, physical health, wealth and spiritual fulfilment – or even just the daily to-do list – life can feel somewhat hectic and repetitive no matter your age or background.

Many people I work with feel as if they are a circus performer, spinning plates or juggling too many balls in the air, waiting in fear for the inevitable crash landing that could happen at any time. As a result, we are stressed – low on humour, fun, compassion, patience, spontaneity and perspective – and this stress builds gradually day-by-day until an uncontrollable feeling of mediocrity infects us to a point of feeling helpless to do anything about it.

Is this as good as it gets?

Underneath our overwhelm lies a deeper fear – *is this as good as it gets?* For many, each birthday with a zero seems to deaden the nerve on our optimism for living an exceptional life. Your 30th, 40th, 50th or 60th birthday may well come along with questions such as: *Is this all there is? Are my best years really behind me?*

Will we ever know true love? Will we ever be appreciated for who we are? Will we ever get our financial house in order and leave the legacy we want? Will we ever find work that we love? Will we ever love our body? Will we ever find true friendship and community? With so many questions unanswered, coupled with an already busy and overwhelming life, it's little wonder so many of us choose the path of least resistance and settle for average in many areas of our lives.

If you relate to any or all of this, I am so glad you're reading this book. We've all been on this path – it's as if we are each destined to set foot on it at some point – and many, sadly, never leave. Tolerating average has become so socially accepted that to plan for an exceptional life can open us to ridicule and rejection.

The risk is that if we stay on the safe path, the long-term consequences of mediocrity can be disastrous.

The consequences of average

Given we're so busy spinning plates, most of us never think about the long-term consequences of settling for average. The daily grind of working a job you don't love ends in major regret, or worse still a chronic disease.

The daily excuse of time and fatigue that stops you from exercising robs you of your vitality and energy in the short-term, but puts you at major risk of chronic disease and a loss of dignity in your final years.

Being too busy to socialise might seem normal at the moment, but when your nest is empty or you've retired, the ensuing social isolation and depression is a recipe for disaster.

Being 'ships in the night' with your partner might seem the only way to survive right now, but what if you feel like strangers to each other in five, 10 or 15 years? Resentment left unchecked breeds a bitterness that often ends in divorce and heartache.

Spending more than you earn might seem the only solution in your current environment, but do you really want to be like 69% of the population and retire on the pension?

If you settle for long-term 'average' in just one area of life, the rest eventually comes tumbling down. Look at any person who ate, smoke or drank themselves sick over many years – and you'll see the eventual impact on the family, finances, health, friendships, spirit and career.

But where do you start on this adventure to exceptional? What if you have many areas of life you want to improve but are unsure where to begin? What if you want to audit your life and are unsure how to measure it? I'm glad you asked. After years of research, investigation and self-analysis, it became clear that *The Exceptionals* live by what I have come to call the Exceptional Life Blueprint.

INTRODUCTION

The Exceptional Life Blueprint

Throughout this book I'll talk about life as a recipe and you as the chef. Think of your Exceptional Life Blueprint as a dish with eight ingredients –

1. Life Purpose/career
2. Movement
3. Social Life
4. Nutrition
5. Family
6. Growth
7. Wealth
8. Spirit

The *order* of which you put each ingredient into your life and the *amount* of each has a major impact. Do you prioritise wealth over family and friends? What happens if you put in too much work and not enough family or nutrition? How does the recipe of life taste if you put family first and your spirit last? I have battled, experimented with and explored these conundrums for years. And finally, here is what I discovered.

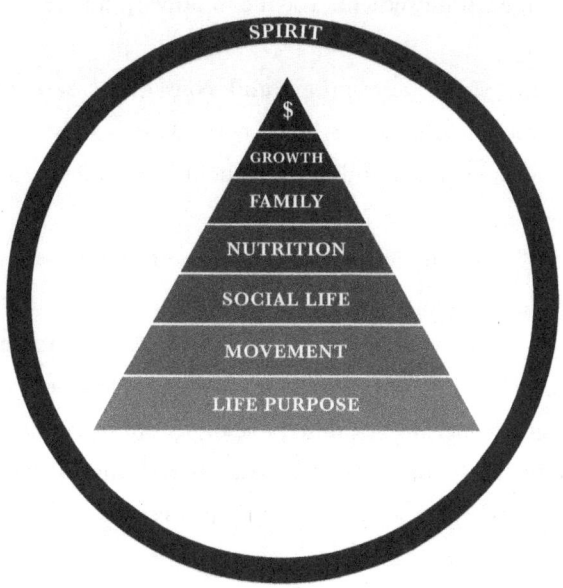

Your longevity or quantity of life is largely determined by three ingredients: your life purpose (career), movement and social life. The quality of your life is most impacted by four ingredients: your nutrition, your family relationships, your growth and your wealth. I call these quality of life enhancers if they are present in your life, or destroyers if they are absent. They may not always add to longevity, but at any age these four ingredients will enrich your life.

There is another essential ingredient, however, and that is spirit. If you avoid putting your spirit – your heart and soul – into each ingredient, your life simply becomes a to-do list of doing the right things, judging your success on your achievements (human *doing*) rather than your fulfilment and who you are as a person (human being).

Exceptional Exercise 0.1: Examine your life

Socrates said "The unexamined life is not worth living." This book is an invitation to examine your life in a way you never have before. Begin by taking a moment to look at the following assessment. Identify where you are in each area of life and give yourself a score out of 10 in each ingredient. You'll end up with a maximum score of 80.

Look at the short descriptions and consequences of mediocre and exceptional to generate your score. This is only a snapshot, and by the time you've finished this book, the numbers are likely to change.

A word of caution here: some readers mark themselves more harshly than others. Personally, an 8/10 or above is exceptional for me. A score of seven and under feels average to me. Each reader will be different, and I ask you to assess your own life accordingly. Generally speaking, five or six out of 10 is considered to be mediocre. It doesn't feel bad enough to change, yet is nowhere near the life that you want. It's simply average.

INTRODUCTION

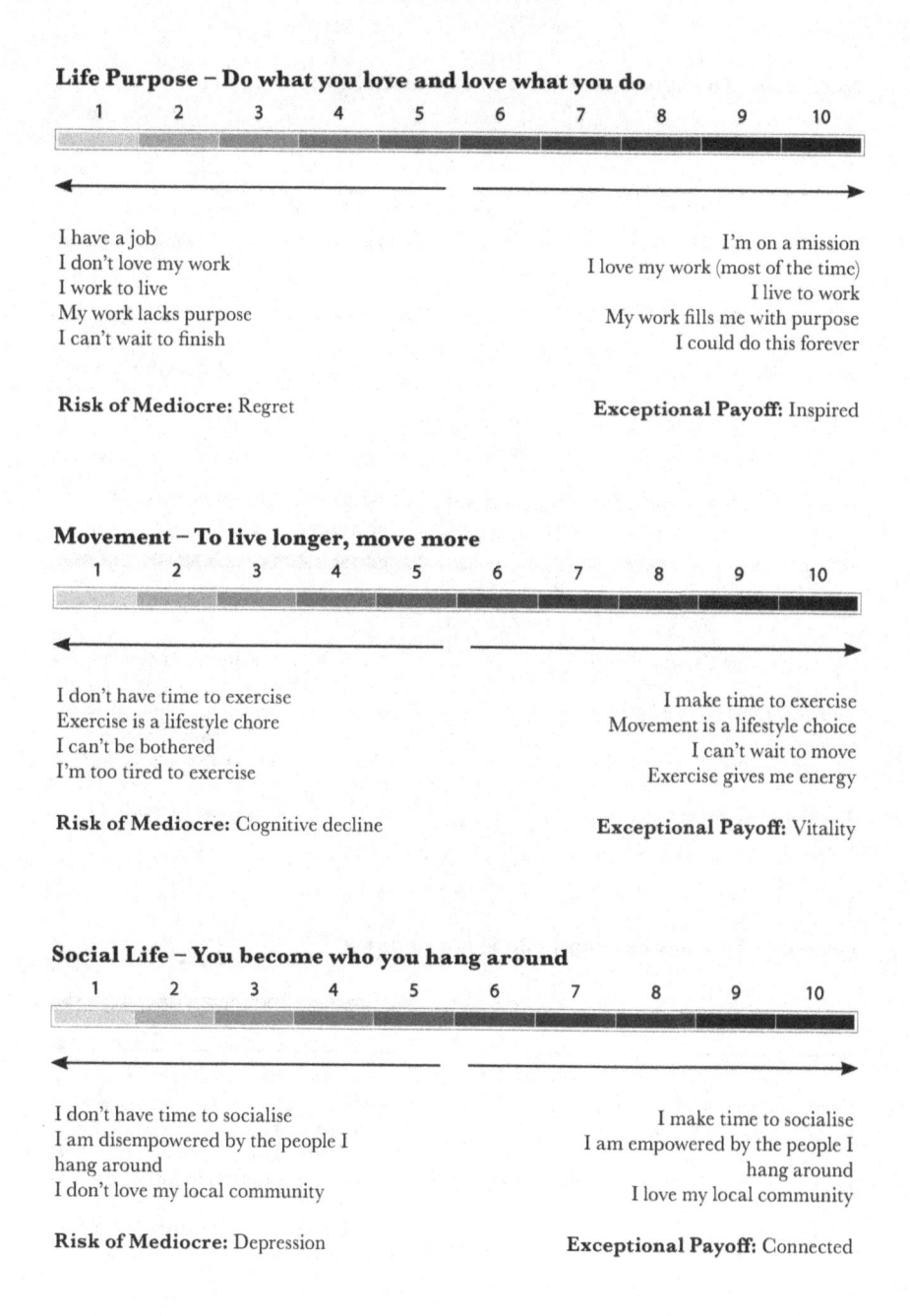

Life Purpose – Do what you love and love what you do

| 1 | 2 | 3 | 4 | 5 | 6 | 7 | 8 | 9 | 10 |

←——————————————————→ ←——————————————————→

I have a job   I'm on a mission
I don't love my work   I love my work (most of the time)
I work to live   I live to work
My work lacks purpose   My work fills me with purpose
I can't wait to finish   I could do this forever

Risk of Mediocre: Regret   **Exceptional Payoff:** Inspired

Movement – To live longer, move more

| 1 | 2 | 3 | 4 | 5 | 6 | 7 | 8 | 9 | 10 |

←——————————————————→ ←——————————————————→

I don't have time to exercise   I make time to exercise
Exercise is a lifestyle chore   Movement is a lifestyle choice
I can't be bothered   I can't wait to move
I'm too tired to exercise   Exercise gives me energy

Risk of Mediocre: Cognitive decline   **Exceptional Payoff:** Vitality

Social Life – You become who you hang around

| 1 | 2 | 3 | 4 | 5 | 6 | 7 | 8 | 9 | 10 |

←——————————————————→ ←——————————————————→

I don't have time to socialise   I make time to socialise
I am disempowered by the people I   I am empowered by the people I
hang around   hang around
I don't love my local community   I love my local community

Risk of Mediocre: Depression   **Exceptional Payoff:** Connected

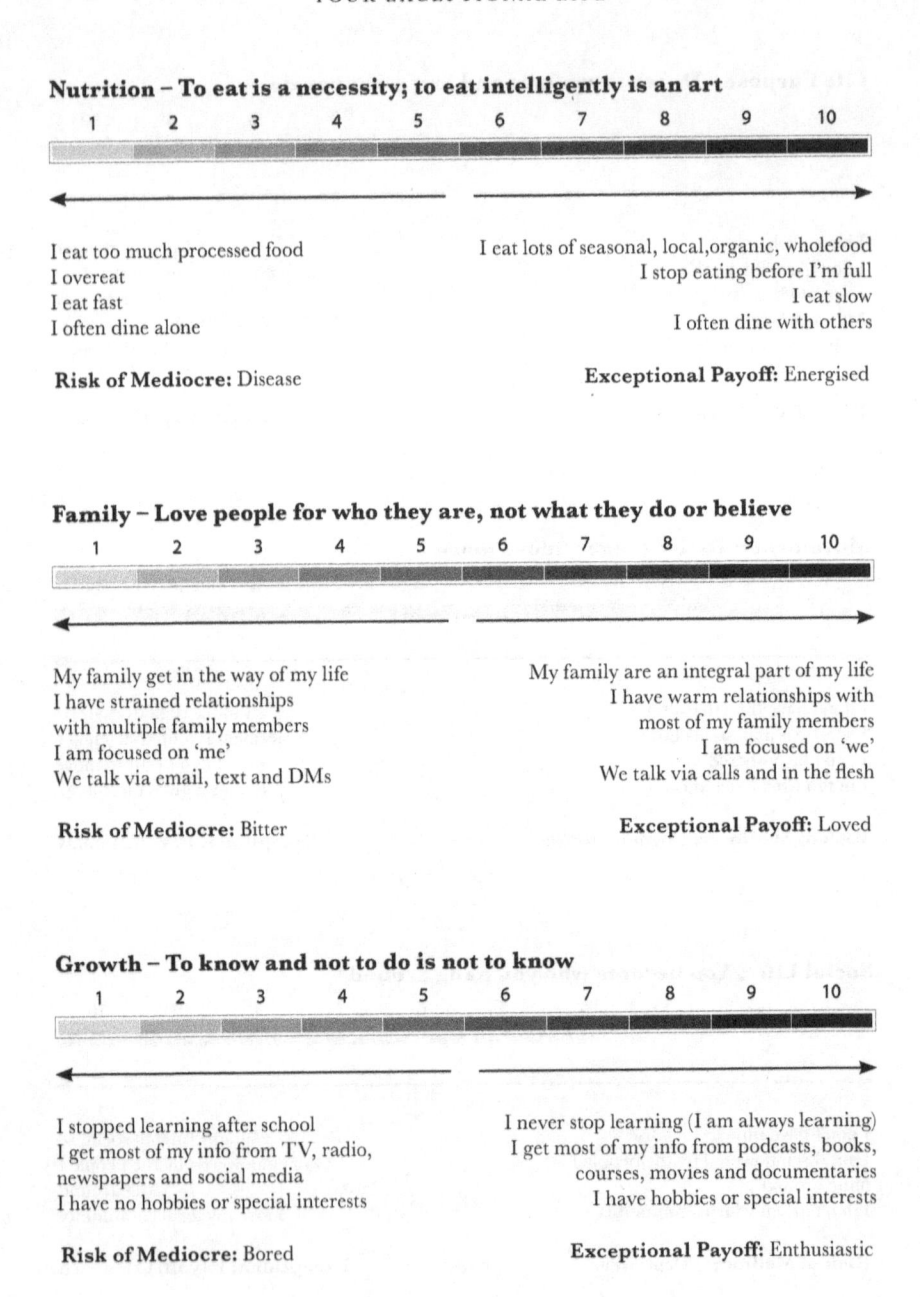

YOUR EXCEPTIONAL LIFE

Nutrition – To eat is a necessity; to eat intelligently is an art

1 2 3 4 5 6 7 8 9 10

I eat too much processed food
I overeat
I eat fast
I often dine alone

Risk of Mediocre: Disease

I eat lots of seasonal, local, organic, wholefood
I stop eating before I'm full
I eat slow
I often dine with others

Exceptional Payoff: Energised

Family – Love people for who they are, not what they do or believe

1 2 3 4 5 6 7 8 9 10

My family get in the way of my life
I have strained relationships
with multiple family members
I am focused on 'me'
We talk via email, text and DMs

Risk of Mediocre: Bitter

My family are an integral part of my life
I have warm relationships with
most of my family members
I am focused on 'we'
We talk via calls and in the flesh

Exceptional Payoff: Loved

Growth – To know and not to do is not to know

1 2 3 4 5 6 7 8 9 10

I stopped learning after school
I get most of my info from TV, radio,
newspapers and social media
I have no hobbies or special interests

Risk of Mediocre: Bored

I never stop learning (I am always learning)
I get most of my info from podcasts, books,
courses, movies and documentaries
I have hobbies or special interests

Exceptional Payoff: Enthusiastic

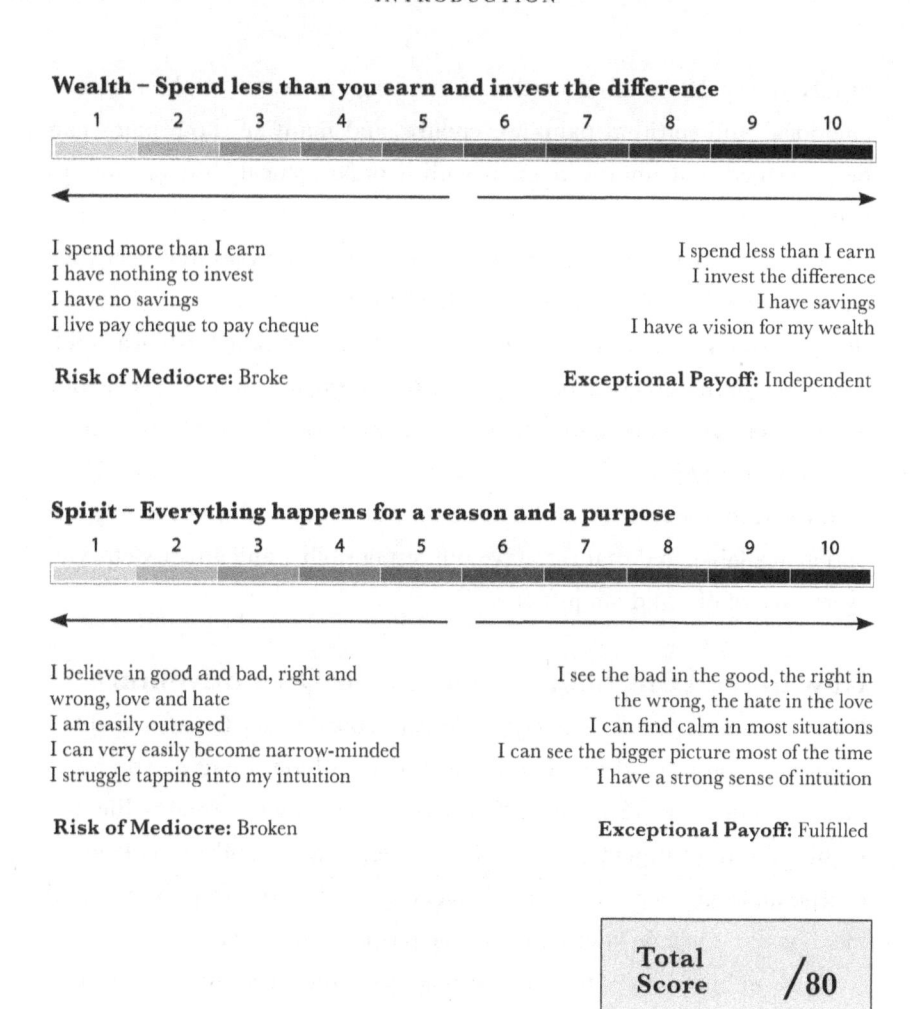

Wealth – Spend less than you earn and invest the difference

1 2 3 4 5 6 7 8 9 10

I spend more than I earn	I spend less than I earn
I have nothing to invest	I invest the difference
I have no savings	I have savings
I live pay cheque to pay cheque	I have a vision for my wealth

Risk of Mediocre: Broke   **Exceptional Payoff:** Independent

Spirit – Everything happens for a reason and a purpose

1 2 3 4 5 6 7 8 9 10

I believe in good and bad, right and wrong, love and hate	I see the bad in the good, the right in the wrong, the hate in the love
I am easily outraged	I can find calm in most situations
I can very easily become narrow-minded	I can see the bigger picture most of the time
I struggle tapping into my intuition	I have a strong sense of intuition

Risk of Mediocre: Broken   **Exceptional Payoff:** Fulfilled

Total Score	/80

Do you choose an exceptional or average life?

Looking at the above table and your scores, how will life turn out if you settle for average in any area of your life? What impact will this decision have on your family, your friends, your work, your wider community, and most importantly, on you?

These future consequences are real and all too common. There is nothing make-believe or fanciful in this book. Whilst I am accused (quite rightly) of being a romantic idealist when it comes to living an exceptional life, may I remind you there is nothing romantic about the consequences of mediocrity. If anything, settling for average gives rise to the physical, emotional and spiritual pains we endure; and many of those pains can be prevented and improved upon with a philosophical shift on how to live life.

I doubt you're reading this right now saying *I choose average*, however your current behaviour and standards in life might say otherwise. Of course, there are times in life where we become out of balance. The birth of a child, a new job, business endeavour or family bereavement will tip the scales for all of us. The key is not to live there forever and make the event a reason for accepting average.

If you want the rest of your life to be the best of your life, there is only one option available, and that is to take full responsibility and go for victory in every area of life, and not just one.

How to read this book: Choose Your Own Adventure

I loved reading *Choose Your Own Adventure* books when I was a child. I encourage you to read this book in a similar fashion. Imagine you are a first responder at a crash scene. Your job is to identify the areas of life that require the most urgent attention first. If your career and movement are exceptional but you're social life is lacking, start at the section on social life. If you're stuck on your career or life purpose, start there.

Keep in mind that the Exceptional Life Blueprint model is not a mountain where wealth is the summit or the peak. Instead, look at it as a triangular jigsaw puzzle, with life purpose being the biggest piece and wealth the smallest. Your spirit is the box that houses your exceptional life.

Part One of this book is dedicated to your longevity and quantity of life. We'll explore your life purpose, movement and social life.

Part Two is dedicated to creating an exceptional quality of life. We look at nutrition, family, growth and wealth.

Part Three is dedicated to unleashing your exceptional spirit by putting your heart and soul into each area of life.

The primary message of the book is that all eight ingredients of your exceptional life are connected to and rely on each other. Your work life impacts your family life, your nutritional choices and your peer group. When you make wise financial decisions, you and your family thrive. When you eat well, you're more present with your work or family. When you move well, you have more energy and vitality to thrive in every other area of life. There is no independence or segmenting of these different components.

Identifying *The Exceptionals*

Anyone in this book who has their year of birth in brackets at their first mention is considered an *Exceptional*. Oprah Winfrey (b. 1954) is, for example, a member of *The Exceptionals*. There are more than 60 *Exceptionals* featured throughout the book. Many direct quotes from *The Exceptionals* have been taken from interviews I have done with them on my podcast, *100 Not Out*. You'll find a complete list of *The Exceptionals* and episode numbers at the back of this book. A selected Bibliography has also been included if you would like to learn more about *The Exceptionals*.

Exceptional Exercises

Each section includes a number of exercises to help you consciously create your exceptional life. These exercises have been compiled into a printable workbook available at **marcuspearce.com.au/yourexceptionallife**. That same website has an array of further learning materials, profiles of *The Exceptionals*, and much more.

Let's begin a lifelong adventure

Manifesting an exceptional life doesn't necessarily happen quickly or easily. You're about to go on a mind and soul-expanding journey through this book that will both challenge and inspire you. The challenge laid down in this book represents a marathon more than a sprint. The average life stretches more than 30,000 days, so tread gently and be kind to yourself. All I ask is that you persevere; living your exceptional life is a journey and not a destination.

As you read this book, avoid comparing yourself to *The Exceptionals* – or anyone for that matter. Instead, let *The Exceptionals* invite and inspire you to rediscover or remind you that you are an exceptional human being. You are one of a kind. Your magnificence has not left you. It may be buried deep down, but it's there, waiting to be recovered. Let the principles, stories and strategies contained in this book propel you forward so that the *rest* of your life truly will be the *best* of your life.

Let's get to work.

> *"Let go of who you're supposed to be; embrace who you are."*
> **– Brené Brown**

PART ONE

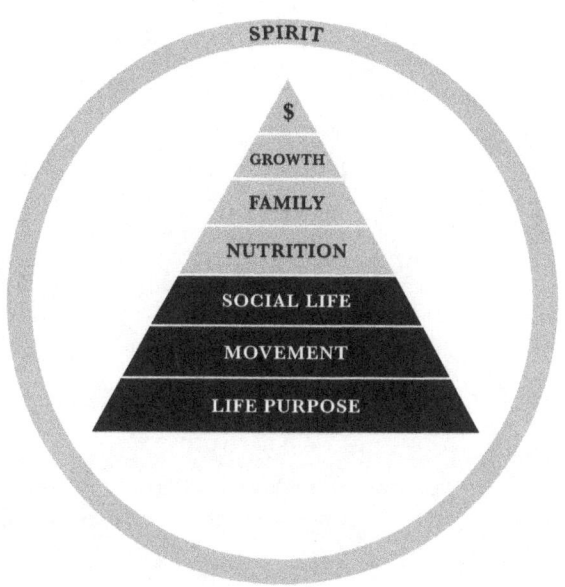

YOUR EXCEPTIONAL
LONGEVITY

YOUR EXCEPTIONAL LIFE

LIFE PURPOSE

"The meaning of life is to find your gift.
The purpose of life is to give it away."
– *Pablo Picasso*

The purpose of your life – the reason you were born to live, your life's task, your calling, your life's work, your dream job, your dhárma or your passion – rarely presents itself on a silver platter.

Perhaps your life's purpose was born out of difficult circumstances. It could be the pains of labour, or major resistance to your career choice from family, a tragedy or crisis with seemingly insurmountable hurdles.

The seed of your life's purpose may be less dramatic. You may have been born with or discovered a magnificent obsession early (or later) in life, or your journey might be to pick up where your parents left off – and achieve what they were not able to achieve.

Your life purpose might be easy to define or it may seem incredibly difficult to articulate. What is true for any *Exceptional* is a yearning or magnetic attraction to live the life you were born to live.

From Florence Nightingale to Leonardo Da Vinci, Richard Branson to Oprah Winfrey and all the *Exceptionals* you've never heard of; you'll find a magnificent life purpose has not been an overnight success, nor has it been an easy ride.

Moreover, your life purpose is not simply about what you do during your working hours. Instead, your *behaviour* and *character* will leave just as much, if not more of a legacy than your achievements. If you're mean, bigoted and judgemental, the people close to you will remember these traits a whole lot more than what you accomplished.

So an exceptional life purpose is not easy. It calls for an unconditional dedication to a standard many in society are not willing to aim for. In order to live your exceptional life purpose you'll need to deal with a never-ending line of fears and challenges. However, knowing that this is the path you have chosen will create a personal resilience you never knew existed.

▲ ▲ ▲

Defying the People We Love the Most

Florence Nightingale's mother and sister were aghast that Florence didn't want to become a wife and mother (the expected role for a woman of her status). Florence instead wanted to devote her life to the service of others, and began by educating herself in the art and science of nursing.

Nepalese ophthalmologist Dr Sanduk Ruit (b. 1954) was told by his parents that his career was to follow in his father's footsteps as a salt trader. Today, having personally brought sight back to over 130,000 human beings, the world's foremost eye surgeon is known as the 'God of Sight'.

Albert Einstein (1879–1955) wanted to dedicate his life to the natural laws of the universe, while his father, Hermann, simply wanted his son to get a steady job.

Defying the important people who believe they are the scriptwriters of your life is not easy. Chances are, they are the same people who raised you, educated you, paid you or loved you. For many, defying these well-meaning scriptwriters is a task so insurmountable that to tolerate mediocrity is a more viable alternative. For *The Exceptionals*, dealing with these opponents is just another step (albeit a significant one) on the path to doing their life's work.

Who are your life purpose opponents?

If any of the aforementioned *Exceptionals* heeded the advice of their well-meaning challengers, you would not be reading about them in this book. What is clear from my research of exceptional human beings is that overcoming someone, or a group of people, who do not believe or share in the same vision you have for your life, is a part of the journey to living your exceptional life purpose.

Who are your life purpose opponents? Who is consciously or subconsciously attempting to stop you realising your dreams?

Is it:

- Your parents who want you to be comfortable and live the life *they* planned for you?
- Your partner who thinks it's too risky to start something new?
- Your siblings who are wary of you being 'better' than them?
- Your boss who thinks you'll fail in a new venture or role?
- Your colleagues who question your ability?
- Your friends who have the same fears as your siblings and fear being left behind?
- The traditional mass media – television, radio and print – who want you to keep your eyes glued to *their* agenda rather than spending time on your agenda?
- Social media 'friends' and influencers who project perfection, success or fame without any substance?

Consciously living *your* exceptional life is akin to leaving the village and tribe who raised you. You'll be hard pressed to find much support, particularly at the beginning. If you still scratch your head when looking for a well-meaning opponent in your life, all you need to do is look in the mirror. *Your* limiting beliefs, *your* negative self-talk, *your* imposter syndrome tendencies, *your* rationalisations to justify your behaviour will often challenge you more than anyone else.

The biggest regret of life

Grace was dying and she knew it. Her family knew it too but dared not to bring it up in conversation. Desperate to express herself and share her final thoughts on life – the highlights, the lowlights, the lessons and the regrets – Grace turned to the palliative carer who would be there for each and every one of the final days of her life. The carer's name was Bronnie Ware (b. 1967), and the major regret Grace shared with Bronnie was: "I wish I'd had the courage to live a life true to myself, not the life others expected of me."[1]

It wasn't 'I wish I'd earned more money' or 'I wish I'd travelled more of the world' or 'I wish I'd spent more time in the office'. Grace's number one regret was the missed opportunity she had to live a truly exceptional life on her own terms; instead she opted for the safe, socially accepted path of doing what would please or satisfy others before herself.

Ware worked as a palliative carer for eight years, spending time with more than 200 dying people in their homes before their life came to an end. She encountered this same regret over and over again. These regrets came to form a very successful book for publisher Hay House. *The Top 5 Regrets Of The Dying* remains one of the publisher's fastest-translated books ever. Why? Because the message of regret struck a chord in humanity, and Ware's book made it urgent for readers to deal with regrets whilst time allowed, instead of facing them on their deathbed.

You are the most important person in your world

I remember it like it was yesterday. It was 2005 and I was a young TV producer looking to quit my job and travel the world. From the outside looking in, I had a job many people dreamed of. It was a job you would *never* quit (because who knows when you would be offered anything like it again) and I was well up the ladder to becoming a highly regarded producer. My wonderful boss and executive producer, Tim, said something to me late one night when I was confiding my thoughts to him and his words have never left my heart. He told me, "You are the most important person in your world."

It's a difficult statement to grasp. Many of us have simply forgotten to consider ourselves as number one. Out of touch with our own needs, desires and dreams, the modern day martyr instead puts children, partners, parents, employers or friends in front of the queue. We get so busy helping everyone else live their exceptional lives that we become too exhausted to live our own.

Consider this metaphor: visualise a jug full of water – its ingredients are your time, energy, love and inspiration. Each day you wake up and it's full. Who has the first sip? For many parents, their children take the first sips. And after school drop off their employer or the house gets the next gulp. And as the day wears on, everyone else is drinking out of the jug of *your* energy, time, love and inspiration. Who is giving the water away? You are. And what happens? After a while the jug is empty and dry. As a result, *you* feel empty and dry too. Bitter, resentful and feeling helpless to turn it all around, over time you find that not only does the jug refuse to refill itself each night, you've lost the art of filling it up yourself.

If the jug metaphor resonates with you, this book will not only help you refill the jug, but also ensure that it is filled up each day and that on rising *you* take the first big sip. When you do this, you give your love, energy, time and inspiration with a full heart, and not an empty one.

If you're already giving from a full jug, this book serves as a reminder to stay on the path, because even the most exceptional people can fall into a pit of mediocrity and chronic self-sacrifice.

The most selfless and loving thing you can do for the people around you and humanity at large is to express yourself and your life to the fullest. This is a beautiful blend of selfish and selfless. But don't just take my word for it. Throughout this book you'll find countless examples of *Exceptionals* who wrote their own script and followed their bliss despite the pushback, pain and harshest of circumstances.

Why We're Confused About Our Purpose in Life

Many of us live our lives in fear of what others will think of us if we go against the grain. When it comes to our career – be it as a parent, self-employed or employee – one of the most passive and soul-destroying ways we limit ourselves is through the toxicity of comparison.

Comparison has always been a part of the human condition. When we lived in villages we compared ourselves to our family and friends. When transport became more accessible, we compared ourselves with people from other villages. As our population swelled, we began to compare ourselves more against our neighbours and colleagues and people from other countries. And as technology has advanced, we can now instantaneously compare ourselves to millions of strangers thanks to the rise of social media.

Comparing ourselves to others can create fear, helplessness and a mindset that believes we'll never be good enough, strong enough, rich enough, supported enough or pretty enough, to do what *The Exceptionals* are doing.

My life purpose allows me to work with some brilliant leaders in the health, wealth and personal growth fields. These leaders are revered for their success and I know thousands of people who compare their own lives to *The Exceptionals* they admire. In the process of comparing, we often forget the individual's hard work – achieved over years, and often decades – especially on social media. How do you capture or portray decades of grit, rejection, heartbreak and the daily grind in a single image or status update?

How do you capture the sacrifice of Australian nutritionist Cyndi O'Meara (b. 1960), who would get up at 4am each morning whilst her children slept, in order to write her best-seller *Changing Habits Changing Lives?* How do you capture the determination of Temple Grandin (b. 1947), who was born autistic and raised in an era where institutionalisation was the preferred medical treatment? Grandin defied societal and medical norms to become a trailblazer in her chosen profession, going on to revolutionise the treatment of animals in slaughterhouses around the world, despite the rejection of her peers.

How do you capture the resolve of international wellness expert Damian Kristof (b. 1973), who grew up in relative poverty in Melbourne's outer suburbs. Kristof did the exceptional and studied not one but two health professions, first becoming a naturopath and then a chiropractor. His breadth of knowledge would go on to see him appointed co-host of one of the first ever empowering weight-loss programs on TV, *Downsize Me!*

Oprah Winfrey, Richard Branson (b. 1950), and anyone else you love and admire were not 'overnight success' stories. Most media tricks us into feeling that the mountain called *Exceptional* is nothing more than overcoming a few cobblestones. When the hard work really starts, it's easy to see why the climb to *Exceptional* has fewer people at the summit than at basecamp. Reality rarely meets expectation when the climb to *Exceptional* is underway.

What you see when you're consuming mainstream media is never the entire truth. Social media is merely one side of the coin – and the side that people want us to know. Think about it for a second – do you pull your camera out and take selfies when you're in a terrible mood, yelling at your children or when your greatest plans are coming undone? I know I don't! Social media is an infinitely small component of reality. And sadly, this tiny component is what billions of people are comparing themselves to.

We are suffering from Facebook envy

The numbers are confronting yet unsurprising. In 2020, 3.8 billion people were using social media, representing 49% of the global population at the time.[2] Over two thirds of American adults use Facebook, which has 2.32 billion active monthly users (i.e they have logged into Facebook in the past 30 days).[3] By generation, 90.4% of Millennials, 77.5% of Generation X and 48.2% of Baby Boomers are active social media users.[4] We spend an average of 2 hours and 22 minutes per day on social media, checking our phones on average 28 times per day.[5]

All of this use causes for many what has been termed 'Facebook envy' – the tendency to be jealous of your friends' activities on social media. Research at the University of Copenhagen on 1095 individuals (86% were female with an average age of 34) revealed that users who took a week-long break from Facebook were found to be more satisfied with life.[6]

What's fascinating (and not all that surprising) is that 13% of the abstainers admitted to giving in and using Facebook due to an emergency or 'habitual accident'.[7] I could replace the word Facebook with Instagram, TikTok, alcohol, cigarettes or any other drug. For many, the addiction to social media is not dissimilar to a drug addiction.

A picture may tell a thousand words but it's never the whole story

On a family trip to Europe in 2018 we passed the biggest field of sunflowers I have ever seen. My wife, Sarah, was spellbound and was determined to get a photo in the field. Not *of* the field or *in front of* the field but *in* the field. No matter that we had three tired children and had spent the day touring regional France; this was one of those moments where, hell or highwater, we *would* get the photo that would last a lifetime and evoke idyllic memories of our family holiday.

The reality was that bees were hovering around the sunflowers. Our son Darby was very concerned that he would be stung by a bee; our youngest and breastfeeding son, Tommy, decided this was the perfect time for some *booby juice*; our oldest child, Maya, was frustrated that she wasn't getting the attention she deserved, whilst Sarah and I were navigating our way through hundreds of five-foot yellow and green sunflowers that were the subject of our angelic family photo.

In spite of all of this, we managed to take a burst of photos and put one of them up on social media to thunderous applause. According to the social media landscape, whether the kids were smiling or not was not important, and whether we were in fact happy or not at this time in our travels was definitely not important. The very fact that it was my most popular photo on Instagram that month is what mattered. Right?

I hope you sense my sarcasm. I'll never know what people thought as a result of seeing the photo. Did they wish they could do what we were doing? Were they jealous that we were in Europe and they were not? Were my so-called followers frustrated that their partner would never financially prioritise a six-week holiday with family? Or were they aware that behind the pop of yellow sunflowers was the mental, emotional and physical challenge of parenting young children on the other side of the planet in a different time zone, different culture, different language and a general greater sense of uncertainty for all involved? Whatever the case, analysing even just one social media post can demonstrate how little we really know of what is going on in someone's life.

Exceptional Exercise 1.1:
Remove the poison that causes life purpose confusion

If you've ever been caught up in comparing yourself to someone on social media, here are three techniques I personally use to remove comparison from my own life.

1. **Go on a social and mass media diet.** Ripping the bandaid off and going on a seven (or even 30) day diet that removes all media will yield clarity you never knew existed. Unplug your TV, delete your social apps and replace mass media with personalised media. Choose from inspiring movies, podcasts *you* want to listen to, and books that make you think and bring out the best in you.

2. **Be genuinely happy for the person in whatever it is they've achieved.** One comment is better than 10 likes. If someone you know has achieved something worthy of your congratulations, comment *sincerely* rather than liking the post and moving on. Tell them how happy you are for them. Better yet, if you know them personally give them a call, send them a message or change the experience from digital to real life.

> **3. Get your fix through online groups.** The most social way to engage in social media is by connecting with like-minded people and actually commenting. Facebook groups, the modern day 'online forum' or club are the most empowering way to use social media because written conversation actually takes place with like-minded people.

The ultimate gift of ditching comparison

When you ditch comparison from your life you spend less time in fear or thinking about what others think of you. As a result, you have far more time to think about *you* and creating the life you were born to live.

Whilst I have a wife and four kids who love me, I know for sure that – outside of myself – not one person on this planet wakes up each morning and dedicates their day to me. Is anyone waking up dedicated to living *your* exceptional life? Are you? If your day begins and ends by dedicating yourself to others and never yourself, I can guarantee you that giving from an empty jug will not fulfil you.

It's *your* responsibility to dedicate your life to the exceptional *you* – to fill *your* jug so that it's overflowing. When you have a surplus of self-love, you can then give the overflow to everyone else because you already have so much for yourself.

When you remove comparison you lower your fear and increase your confidence. With that in mind, you're ready to take the five big steps to an exceptional life purpose.

▲ ▲ ▲

Five Steps to Live Your Life's Work

Before you get overwhelmed (as so many people do when attempting to discover their life's work), I want you to consider your life's work as only the next one to seven years of your life – not your entire life. There is a magic about seven-year cycles which I'll explain later in this chapter, and you may be in the middle of one now. As a result, you may feel comfortable only looking towards the next three years or so.

If you're expecting your first child whilst reading this, your life's purpose is about to undergo an incredible transformation. It's difficult to clarify life purpose in the middle of such change. If you're just about to retire, you might want to consider the next seven years, or perhaps just the next 12 months. Whatever your individual circumstance, choose a time frame you feel comfortable with.

There is a worksheet available at **marcuspearce.com.au/yourexceptionallife** to guide you through this five-step process.

Step 1: Identify the seeds of your life's work

The first step to live your life's work is to identify what experiences have taken place in your life. This step requires you to examine your life, and spend the necessary time doing so. When you look deeply at your past and present life, you'll find clues and blessings in disguise hiding behind life experiences you never thought meant all that much. Synchronicities, convenient coincidences and I-couldn't-have-done-it-if-I-tried moments often have a hidden power that we are unable to appreciate for the gifts they are because we don't examine our lives enough.

As you read the examples in the coming pages, you will begin to see the clues life has been whispering to you as to what your life is dedicated to. If you already know what your life's task is, the following will simply confirm it to you. This section requires an open mind and heart to see how some of your biggest challenges have been the seeds of your exceptional life.

The eight seeds of an exceptional life purpose

The path to discovering and living out your life's work is akin to sprinkling seeds in soil. Some life experiences will sprout and leave lasting impressions on you. Others will fail to thrive and disappear into the unconscious, never to be brought up again. Often in life, the experiences we least expect to impact us are the ones that wield incredible influence.

Each seed represents the varied experiences you've had in life that in reality are secrets or clues to what your daily life is dedicated to. You may have experienced tragedy and crisis, resistance from people around you, family pressure to succeed, or an obsession or burning desire you simply can't shake. These are just some of the seeds which, if allowed to sprout, combine to become your purpose in life. As you read them, tick off or make a note of the ones which exist in your life.

Seed 1: Resistance

In just four generations we have seen rapid change in the influence of parents on children and their career choices. Only 100 years ago, it was almost exclusively the domain of the father to choose the career choice of his children, with the boys likely to follow in their dad's footsteps and the girls trained to become refined women, housewives and eventually mothers. How times have changed! Today we are encouraged to follow our dreams rather than simply follow in the footprints of our parents.

This is, however, not the case for all of us. Our desire to win the love and respect of our parents by being 'successful' in life is often not as simple as it seems. The *success* of getting married, having children, starting a business or winning a job of status are uniquely intertwined in a race for our parents love and approval.

An exceptional vision or goal though is often met with resistance from the people closest to you, particularly parents (and often domineering father figures) and colleagues. Historic examples include Einstein and Mozart, but there are numerous modern day *Exceptionals* who have had to overcome significant resistance from parents. Ruth Bader Ginsburg (1933–2020), social justice lawyer and champion of gender equality studied law at Harvard before finishing at Columbia Law School, graduating equal first in her class. Her entire profession shunned her because she was a woman. Finding it nigh on impossible to get a job in the law, Ginsburg spent more than a decade as an academic before co-founding the Women's Rights Project in 1972. In 1993, Ginsburg was appointed as an associate justice of the Supreme Court, where she served until her death in 2020.

> *"My mother told me to be a lady. And for her, that meant be your own person, be independent."*
> **– Ruth Bader Ginsburg**

We love our son, but he's crazy!

Paulo Coelho (b. 1947) is the author of *The Alchemist*, what Oprah Winfrey calls "the book of the century". Coelho fought against major family resistance to become a writer.

"First, they tried to bribe me (to give up on writing)," recalled Coelho in a *SuperSoul Conversations* interview with Winfrey.[8] "Then (they tried) a psychiatrist. Then one day they lost hope and they said 'this guy is crazy. Our son – we love him – but he's crazy'."

Coelho's parents thought their son was crazy because he wasn't conforming to the societal expectations of becoming an engineer, lawyer or other high-ranking employee. Coelho wanted to be an artist. "(My parents' view of artists were) – 'oh, they starve to death, they drink, they do everything that our middle class, affluent family can't stand,'" Coelho said.

Coelho's parents decided to enrol him in a psychiatric institution, not once but three times. Each time, Coelho escaped. "They didn't put me there out of hatred," Coelho reflected to Winfrey. "They were trying to help me. They really thought that I was crazy." Thankfully, Coelho defied his family to arguably become the author of the 21st century with an estimated 350 *million* books sold around the globe.

Seed 2: Born or married into it

It seems some people get a head start in life because they are born into a profession. My dentist, for example, is a fifth generation dentist. You may be a third generation teacher or motor mechanic, farmer or lawyer. Whatever the case may be, being born into or married into a profession can have a significant bearing on your career choice.

If you choose to follow a different career path to your family, the seed of resistance often comes into play.

Seed 3: Exposure to the opposite

The life you were born to live may be close to the exact opposite of what you were exposed to growing up – and the reason for that exposure is to clarify and solidify in your heart and soul what you do *not* want for your life, and perhaps for others as well.

If you grew up in poverty, it's quite common to have a desire for wealth. If you were raised in a violent household, you are likely to want to provide calm and peace in the home. The unstable parts of your upbringing are often the highest priorities for 'correction' in your own adult life.

Children often discover this when they become parents for the first time. All the parenting methods you were exposed to (which you didn't like or don't agree with) become the opposite of how you raise your children. If you were raised in a 'children should be seen and not heard' family culture and you resent it, you're likely to give your children more latitude and freedom. Furthermore, you're likely to give your children what you didn't receive when you were younger.

My grandfather was an alcoholic who was absent as a parent, and my dad despised him for it. Whatever my grandfather would have done, my dad did the opposite. Dad rarely drinks (I've never seen him drunk) and loves to spend time with his children and grandchildren. The pain of Dad's upbringing was a seed of his life purpose, and thankfully my sisters and I were the recipients of the lessons my grandfather bestowed on his son.

No matter how *opposing* your upbringing was to your beliefs of the ideal childhood, remember that we only get the challenges we can handle, and sometimes those challenges are there to show us how *not* to behave when we are in similar circumstances.

Seed 4: Your parents didn't quite make it or gave up on their dreams

Before he was conscripted to serve in the Vietnam War, Normie Rowe (b. 1947) was dubbed Australia's 'King of Pop'. In a twist of fate not dissimilar to his mother's, Rowe's career was impacted by global war. "As a little kid my mum was always singing," Rowe shared with me on *100 Not Out*. "She came from a family of 11 or 12 kids. She always went to the May Downs dancing school, which still exists today. I think had it not been for the end of the First World War and into the Depression and the Second World War, Mum or some of her sisters may have ended up being dancers or singers of some sort. We rarely had a Saturday night where there wasn't some sort of music, joy, happiness, singing and general fun and laughter and a gregarious outgoing lifestyle."

Growing up watching his parents sing and entertain at family gatherings, Rowe developed a magnificent obsession with music and performance. He became the first Australian artist to ever have two top three singles simultaneously for three consecutive weeks and went on to support Roy Orbison in the US and represented Australia alongside The Seekers at Expo '67 in Montreal.

Seed 5: Family desire for fame, wealth or success

A derivative of the parent who didn't make it is the family quest for fame, wealth or (cultural measures of) success. Child prodigies often fall into this category. Many professional artists and sportspeople sprout from this seed, and it can be sowed by parents who want their children to have more opportunities than they did. Parents with low-paying jobs often want their children to seek higher-paying professions. Immigrant families are renowned for working incredibly hard in order to finance their children's education or pathway into a life of greater opportunity.

Like many before him and many after him, tennis icon Andre Agassi (b. 1970) grew up in a family where his father Mike dictated and defined what career each child would have. In his autobiography *Open*, Agassi recounts his self-talk as a seven-year-old. "I hate tennis, hate it with all my heart, and still I keep playing, keep hitting all morning, and all afternoon, because I have no choice."[9]

Parents desperate for fame, wealth or success seem to have an innate knowledge of the 10,000 hour rule (explained later in this section), and they drill it in to their children without any conscious care for the child's overall wellbeing. The seven-year-old Agassi would hit 2500 balls per day, 17500 per week. Over the course of a year that's almost one million balls. Of his father, the young Andre observed that Agassi Snr "believes in math. Numbers, he says, don't lie. A child who hits one million balls each year will be unbeatable."[10]

Mike Agassi was right. His son became close to unbeatable *on* the tennis court, winning eight career Grand Slam tournaments. His deeds *on* the court would inspire millions of people around the planet. Life *off* court for Agassi was certainly no Grand Slam victory. He dealt with physical and mental health challenges, relationship breakups and financial crises. Among his litany of speed bumps, Agassi turned to crystal methamphetamine during a career low point in 1997. That same year, his marriage to actress Brooke Shields was in a sharp decline and he had lost all love for his life purpose, the sport of tennis.

The gifts to the world from *The Exceptionals* raised by parents desperate for fame, wealth or success cannot be argued. Each *Exceptional* leaves an incredible legacy to their profession and fans, but the price they have paid in order to share their gifts to the world can be difficult to justify, given the significant mental, emotional, familial, spiritual and often physical burden they have had to endure.

> *"Your children are not your children.*
> *They come through you but not from you and*
> *though they are with you yet they belong not to you."*
> **– Khalil Gibran**

Seed 6: Magnificent obsession

Alice Herz-Sommer (1903–2014) grew up in Prague surrounded by family and friends who loved the arts. Alice's older sister Irma taught her how to play the piano, and Alice developed a magnificent obsession that would go on to save her life.

"My world is music. I am not interested in anything else. Music is so beautiful," proclaimed Alice at age 109 in the Academy Award winning documentary *The Lady In Number Six*.[11] "Beethoven – he is a miracle. His music is not only melody. What is inside (pointing inwards), how it's felt, it is full, it's intensive, it is a mystery. When the music starts, it goes straight away into our souls. We should thank Bach, Beethoven, Brahms, Schubert, Schumann, (for) they gave us beauty, indescribable beauty."

Alice was married to Leopold in 1931, had a son Raphael in 1937, and was a renowned concert pianist across Europe before the Nazis took over Prague in 1938.

At age 39, Alice and Raphael were held prisoner in Theresienstadt, a feeder camp for Auschwitz, and the place where the Nazi's kept the Jewish intellectuals and artists in order to use them for their own propaganda campaign. Starving prisoners were allowed to compose and give concerts. Alice would go on to play over 100 concerts, playing all 27 of Chopin's Études from memory among a wide-ranging repertoire.

"I felt that music was the only thing which helped me to have hope," recalled Alice. "It is a sort of religion, actually. Music is God."[12]

And perhaps a magnificent obsession is laced with divine intervention. The Holocaust is filled with stories of survival thanks to a valuable career. Herz-Sommer's decision to dedicate her life to music certainly saved her from the gallows, and she is not alone. The oldest survivor of the Holocaust is Yisrael Kristal (1903–2017), whose career as a master confectioner saved his life – for even the Nazis had a sweet tooth.

Seed 7: Higher calling

The definition of call is to 'summon loudly'. A calling is often a summoning from some other source that simply cannot be ignored. Mother Teresa's (1910–1997) calling came through the poverty she witnessed in Calcutta whilst she was a schoolteacher. Domestic violence campaigner Rosemary Batty's calling came after her 11-year-old son, Luke, was murdered by his father.

A higher calling doesn't need to feel religious; it can simply be an unstoppable magnetism to complete a mission or purpose that you may not have chosen consciously. You see a higher calling play out regularly with parents who have children that go through major health challenges, trauma or even death. Others experience a perceived gross injustice and this event becomes the trigger for living a more meaningful life.

Seed 8: Tragedy or crisis

There are no less than eight forms of crisis that may be the powerful seed of your purpose in life. Internal crises – ones that impact you and the close network of people around you – include a family death, divorce, permanent physical injury or chronic health conditions. Business or financial upheavals may be the seed of your life purpose, whilst a social or community crisis (such as public health or crime) is often the bridge to an external crisis.

You may live in a culture or have a faith that has experienced significant challenge, or government policy of some kind may have created upheaval in your life. Many external crises are often cultural, political and religious concurrently, and they then cause internal crises such as financial ruin, poor health or community collapse.

Internal Crises	External Crises
Family	Cultural
Health	Political
Financial or Business	Religious
Social or Community	Environment

A brush with death is a fertile seed for purpose in life

The life's work of Dr Sanduk Ruit was presented to him in the form of a family crisis after his younger sister, Yangla, died at 15. Yangla was the third sibling of Ruit's to die. Her death from tuberculosis was medically preventable, and it was only through a lack of finances that she couldn't be kept alive. It was then, as he shared with me on *100 Not Out*, that Ruit decided to become a doctor.[13]

"I said, 'why does a person like my sister die because of a lack of appropriate medical care. There must be hundreds of thousands of people just like Yangla who are in a similar situation.' This really opened up my belief that this (medicine) is probably the profession that I should get myself into. That was the inspiration and determination I took from Yangla's death. I resolved that I would try everything to get into medicine, and I was successful."

Not only was Ruit successful in becoming a doctor, he would go on to become the first Nepalese ophthalmologist and one of the world's most renowned eye surgeons. On a mission to end preventable blindness in his lifetime, Ruit has personally restored sight to over 130,000 people in developing nations and eye surgeons from all around the world fly to Nepal to learn his methods.

Ruit views the crises he has faced as blessings. "I consider these (crises) as landmarks in my life. Once in a while I go for a short trek up in the mountains. When you reach the top of the hill you have all the time to yourself. You have emptied yourself and you are so fresh to think about some things. I reflect back and I very often think about these landmarks and I say that if these things had not happened – if I had not had such a tough childhood, and if my father didn't have a vision to send me to school, and if I was a 'normal' kid in school and never learnt how to struggle in life. If I didn't lose my sister who was so close to me, would I be doing what I'm doing now?"

Malala Yousafzai (b. 1997) is a trailblazer for female education. The strength of Malala's life purpose only intensified when she was shot in the head by a member of the Taliban whilst on the school bus in her small

Pakistani village – and survived. The physical crisis she experienced as a result of the social, political and religious crisis she endured placed her in the hearts of millions around the world and only added to her power and influence around the globe. In 2014, Yousafzai was awarded the Nobel Peace Prize at age 17, becoming the youngest Nobel Laureate in the award's history.

Turia Pitt's (b. 1987) life purpose was born after a physical and spiritual crisis. Pitt suffered first-degree burns to 65% of her body during the ill-fated fires in the Kimberley region of Australia in 2011. Today, Pitt's life purpose is dedicated to inspiring people through her own resilience and forward-thinking approach to life.

Eddie Jaku's life purpose was sowed in the seed of the Holocaust, a political, cultural, social, family, physical, financial and religious crisis. Today Eddie teaches and inspires humanity to cleanse themselves of hate.

Life can be so brutal

The truth is you may be forced to bury your soul mate or child. You'll farewell friends and your business life will end. Your treasured possessions will break or may burn to a crisp in a few hours. Death, as much as we attempt to deny it, is an essential part of life. Every element of our life will be with us for only a part of our entire life, with one exception: our own life purpose.

Your life purpose is part of your spirit. It is immortal, as it impacts, influences or ripples into other people's lives in a way that you may never know. Whilst it may feel like purpose can end in dramatic circumstances (you get the sack, your business goes under, your marriage ends, a major tragedy strikes), when the dust settles, all that remains is the quest to define what's next.

During crisis, many of us refuse to redefine the next chapter of our exceptional life, largely because of fear and the social belief that it is too indulgent to move on. On the other hand *The Exceptionals* give grace for the people in their past and walk courageously into a new future, no matter how scary and uncertain it may be. As much as you are the scriptwriter of *Your Exceptional Life*, life demonstrates that there is a co-writer – God,

Mother Nature, Buddha, Gaia, Muhammad or whatever you like to call the energy that runs the universe.

Particularly when death strikes, this understanding (also known as faith) that you are not walking the path alone will bind you to an inner belief that this higher power makes no mistakes and as painful as it is, there is a greater cause or purpose to the tragedy.

🔺 🔺 🔺

Step 2: Combine the seeds

It's unlikely that your life purpose sprouted from just one of these eight seeds. Chances are, just like plants thrive in the presence of other companion plants, one of your life purpose seeds has had a companion or two. Wolfgang Amadeus Mozart (1756–1791) had the seed of a magnificent obsession, accompanied by a family upbringing dominated by music and a father who vehemently resisted his son's desire to be a composer. All of this pressure is perhaps what created the diamond that was Mozart.

David Attenborough (b. 1926) knew from the age of eight that he wanted to spend his time studying the natural world. His magnificent obsession combined with the multiple environmental crises Attenborough has identified during his career has only made his work more important – and more respected.

The more I research *The Exceptionals* the more I find resistance from at least one key individual at the heart of a magnificent obsession manifesting itself; it is almost a rite of passage that the universe places in front of us. You have to *fight* for your life purpose against challenges in order to test and define how committed you really are to living your exceptional life.

Embrace the twists of fate and sliding doors

I grew up with a magnificent obsession for Australian rules football, the son of a father who came close to playing at the highest level but never quite made it. Those two seeds sprouted within me for two decades, and when I realised I would not be a great footballer, I decided I would be a

...list and work in the sports media. As luck or fate would have it, the ...y crisis of my parents marriage led to my dad selling his newsagency business and getting a job with a major Australian newspaper.

This media connection allowed me to obtain one week of work experience with the *Herald Sun* sports department when I was 16, and the seed of my life purpose definitely sprouted and roots began to form. Fast forward three years and my mum's partner at the time, Justin, had a friend who worked in sales at a Melbourne sports radio station, Sport 927. I did another week of work experience there, and as a twist of fate would have it, a senior breakfast radio producer resigned not long after my stint. His assistant was promoted and I slotted in to becoming a radio producer at the age of 19.

In a reflection of *Sliding Doors* (that great movie starring Gwyneth Paltrow), I often wonder how my professional life would have turned out if my parents had not split up. When I think of the opportunities and lessons I have had as a result of my parents divorce, it's easy for me to say that their decision to split was the best decision they ever made. My marriage would not be what it is today without the exposure to the opposite I witnessed growing up and my professional life may have turned out completely differently had my parents stayed together. I share my own example and those of *The Exceptionals* as an invitation to you to assess where the seeds of your life purpose live.

Exceptional Exercise 1.2:
Identify the seeds of your life purpose

1. Identify the seeds. Review the eight seeds of your exceptional life purpose and write down specific examples from your own life. Have you had a health crisis, a financial crisis or parents resisting your magnificent obsession? Did you or the people around you quash a childhood passion because you could never see a career in it? Does your gift to the world lie somewhere in the greatest challenges you have gone through?

> 2. Join the seeds. What do these life experiences mean for you? How do they impact your beliefs and subsequent decisions and actions?

Remember, these are *seeds* of your purpose in life, and they may not have been given an opportunity to sprout and grow just yet. This book may be just the beginning of the acorn turning into the oak tree.

Identifying the seeds of your purpose in life may give you clarity and perhaps even some excitement. Clarity however will not deliver you overnight success. Whilst clarity is undoubtedly powerful, it's not enough to guarantee success of any kind. The seed needs *time* to grow.

Step 3: Commit the time

When you have the clarity of what your life purpose is committed to, and the confidence to make it happen, the only barrier remaining is time. As paradoxical as it sounds, the greatest barrier – time – is the only pathway. Society is rife with 'I don't have time' statements. 'I don't have time to exercise', 'I don't have time to catch up with my friends', 'I don't have time to meditate', 'I don't have time to study' and 'I don't have time to be healthy' are commonplace and all socially acceptable statements.

If you're to truly master your life purpose and live your exceptional life, you must be prepared to dedicate *significant* time to its attainment. Many people believe they don't have time to identify their life's purpose, whilst *The Exceptionals* believe as Picasso did, that: "The meaning of life is to find your gift. The purpose of life is to give it away." Put another way, you were born with an incredible gift to give away. Your number one priority is to dedicate the time to discovering exactly what that gift is.

The seven-year apprenticeship leads to overnight success

Every *Exceptional* you admire has been an apprentice to a mentor or master. Robert Greene beautifully outlines the power of spending quality and quantity time learning from a mentor in his book *Mastery*. Leonardo da Vinci (1452–1519) spent over 10 years with the artist Verrocchio, seven of them as his apprentice. Health professionals complete a five-year university degree and ideally the early part of their professional life is viewed as the final chapter in the apprenticeship. Building and other trade apprenticeships around the world last between one and seven years, with apprentices required to complete between 2000 and 12000 work hours before earning certification. Any creation of great quality requires quantity time – a human being, an exceptional relationship, a thriving business, a successful career, skill or a work of art.

"Give me the child for the first seven years and I will give you the man," said St Ignatius Loyola. So many of us in our adult lives are dealing with problems that stem back from our childhood and, by extension, the behaviours of our parents in our first seven years of life.

By design, a parent's mentors are their own parents, aunties, uncles and grandparents. In modern times though, this is rarely the case; sadly not many of us view our elders as mentors. Regardless, if you are determined to master anything in your life, you must have a mentor for a significant period of time.

On the same day that Bronnie Ware gave birth to her daughter, Elena, a publishing contract came through for *The Top Five Regrets Of The Dying* that very quickly spread its wings into 29 different languages. Deemed an overnight success, what wasn't often explained was that Ware had quit her job as a bank manager in order to, in her own words, "look for a job with meaning". That job was as a palliative carer, which she worked at for *eight* years, looking after over 200 dying people (her mentors) in their homes. That career change wasn't meaningful just for Bronnie and her dying patients; it has gone on to inspire millions of people around the planet.

Every master was once an apprentice, and every apprentice has a mentor

Who are your mentors right now? Who has walked the path you intend to walk down? Mentors of today don't necessarily have to be people you know personally. You can immerse yourself in someone's teachings from anywhere on the planet. I do think having a mentor who you can have one-on-one time with, to ask questions of, and get personalised feedback from, is far more powerful.

My personal experience has been that working for mentors for free (or even paying them for the privilege of working with them) is incredibly powerful and provides added accountability to succeed. Do work experience, offer your time for no charge; just do whatever it takes to be in the proximity of *The Exceptionals* and you'll see living proof that we become who we hang around.

The power of seven-year cycles

The seven-year apprenticeship is not a random number plucked by society. If you've experienced a 'seven-year itch' in your life you'll have an understanding of what the passage of time can bring. The number seven has dominated history across all cultures, from ancient wisdom and traditions to modern-day science. Starting off as the number of days it took to create the world (according to Christianity), the number seven appears over 700 times in the Bible. There are seven planets visible to the naked eye, seven chakras, seven heavens in Islam and ancient Judaism, seven deadly sins and seven heavenly virtues.

There are seven colours in a rainbow, seven unique notes in a common musical scale, and the moon's four distinct phases each take approximately seven days to complete. The female body develops in seven-year cycles according to Traditional Chinese Medicine (men are slower with an eight-year cycle), while the human body replaces every single cell over the course of seven years.

Agreeing with the concept of seven-year cycles is not important. What's essential is honouring the *time* it takes to transform and graduate from *apprentice* to *master* in your chosen career. Whether you choose to master

...g, law, gardening or surfing, no seven-day short course or seven-...loma is going to create a shortcut to mastery. The number is seven years and no less.

The Greatest Showman: A seven-year success story

Director Michael Gracey was in Japan shooting a television advertisement for Lipton Ice Tea. The star of the ad was Hugh Jackman (b. 1968), and the pair – who had never met – struck up an instant friendship and mutual respect that led to Jackman sharing with Gracey his dreams for a Hollywood musical movie blockbuster called *The Greatest Showman*, based on the life of circus entertainer P.T. Barnum.

"For the first three years I was acting like I knew the film was going to happen but I really wasn't sure," Jackman recalled at the Sydney premiere of the film. "At the time I'd never done a movie musical, I'd done a lot of movies and a lot of musicals and I'd just hosted the Oscars. I thought 'I'd love to give it a go' but I wasn't sure I'd get a shot."

Not only did Jackman 'get a shot', *The Greatest Showman* went on to become the third highest-grossing musical of all time, taking in a cool US$435 million at the box office. And how long did *The Greatest Showman* take from conception to release? You guessed it – seven years.

Exceptional Exercise 1.3: Your next seven years

Research in the 1990s by K. Anders Ericsson and associates at Berlin's Academy of Music demonstrated that the more we practise the closer we get to achieving mastery in a chosen field.[14] From elite athletes to musicians, teachers to artists, plumbers and professionals you've never heard of, the magic number of hours popularised by Malcolm Gladwell in *Outliers* is 10,000. For some that might be 40 hours per week over five years, for others it might be 20 hours per week for 10 years. Whilst not an exact science by any means, if you're looking for a shortcut on the seven-year-

> apprenticeship, it seems knocking over 10,000 hours as quickly as possible is the answer.
>
> What are you prepared to dedicate seven years or 10,000 hours to? Are you prepared to dedicate 10,000 hours to raising your children, learning aerodynamics, fashion, medicine, history, the piano, archaeology, social justice, international politics or the arts? My first 10,000 hours (1999–2006) were dedicated to journalism in the sports media. My next 10,000 hours were dedicated to the wellness industry (2007–2014) and I'm currently dedicated to helping humanity create exceptional lives. Given that your average life spans more than 700,000 hours, you can master multiple fields in just one lifetime.

Everyday Exceptionals: A word for the parents

My wife Sarah spent five years studying chiropractic and spent a further 12 years in practice before she decided to dedicate her time to being a stay-at-home mum.

"For me personally, when I tried to be a working parent, I felt like I was failing as a mother and failing my clients because my heart now lay elsewhere," recalls Sarah. "I would leave my children with my mum or Marcus, my heart in my throat every time and crying all the way to work."

One night in 2013 Sarah was in tears. Struggling emotionally with the conflict of having dedicated almost 30,000 hours of her life to her profession, my angel was now seriously contemplating the idea of transitioning out of chiropractic and putting all her energy into raising our children. In short, she wanted to reach 10,000 hours with the children sooner rather than later.

"So much of my identity came from being a chiropractor. I wasn't sure I could live life as a stay-at-home mother. I was also burning myself out by trying to do everything, to be today's modern supermum. Everyone else seemed to be able to do it (or so I thought). And yet, the universe sent me a pretty strong repetitive message. So many of my female patients, from young to old said a similar thing when I showed them their health results. Dismayed, sad, and frustrated they would often say, 'I wish I'd taken care of myself earlier. I wish I hadn't put everyone else's needs first'.

"It was this common theme that gave me the courage to walk away from my profession and be the best example I could for my children. I didn't want them seeing me sacrificing myself at the expense of everyone else. And I wanted to be there to watch them grow, especially when they were little. I wanted to be fully present with them, to give them all of my love and focus without distraction. I wanted to be able to do it at a more relaxed pace that was healthier for me, and to still have time to carve out self-care for me and quality time with Marcus. Raising four children is the toughest thing I have ever done, but deciding to do it without the added stress of a career has been one of the best decisions I have ever made for my life."

If you're a stay-at-home parent, know that your current career or purpose in life is largely dedicated to your children. And, if you view your purpose as Rose Kennedy (1890–1995), matriarch of the famous Kennedy clan did, you'll see your life is dedicated to raising a family of world leaders. That doesn't mean your children need to be the next leaders of the free world; instead it means you're raising your children to be valuable members of society, contributing their individual gifts to humanity which ideally you have encouraged and empowered them to share.

On the flipside, your role as a parent may have you now feeling determined to start the business you've always put off, or you may simply want to balance your family time with a part-time job. Whether you're the parent who craves staying at home, whether you're starting a business or re-entering the workforce, you must follow these intuitive hunches – no matter how illogical they seem – in order to live your exceptional life.

And whilst 10,000 hours may seem like a long time, when you do what you love and love what you do, that number not only excites you, you wish you could spend even more time doing it. Which is why the notion of retirement is so preposterous to *The Exceptionals*.

▲ ▲ ▲

Step 4: Never retire

Charles Eugster (1919–2017), a retired dentist who went on to become the fastest man over 95 years of age, described retirement to me as "a financial catastrophe and a health calamity".

"Retirement is voluntary or involuntary unemployment," Eugster shared on *100 Not Out*. "And unemployment is something that is extremely dangerous for your health. Most people after retirement are sick! The statistics from the US show that 92.2% of people over 65 have one or more chronic diseases. We are destroying old age!"

Eugster's point is well made. My home country of Australia sits fourth on the longevity ladder (with a life expectancy of 83 years) yet plummets down to 15th for *quality* of life. Australians on average have 72 quality years and 11 terrible years – over 4000 days – of poor quality of life.[15]

Eugster wasn't simply pontificating about ageing gracefully. I interviewed Eugster twice on *100 Not Out*, and both times he was determined to champion the importance of working. "I practised dentistry until I was 75. When I was 58 I started a dentist newsletter which I continued until I was 82," he told me, "and at that particular time my wife had died and I wasn't feeling particularly good. I thought that I would only live until I was 85 and so I got rid of the publication which was a huge mistake! After that I was unemployed for eight years, which didn't do me any good at all. I managed to find employment again at the age of 90 until 92 for a fitness group. Today I am an author trying to write a book." Eugster went on to release *Age Is Just A Number* in 2017 before dying a few months later from heart failure, aged 97.

"I want to change the world," he told me. "I want to make old age into one of the most fabulous, extraordinary, wonderful, beautiful, glorious, stupendous periods of everybody's life."

In 'retirement', Eugster would go on to win over 100 rowing events, bodybuilding competitions, 36 Masters gold medals, set world records in athletics in distances from 60m to 400m, present an inspiring TEDx talk and become a published author. Not a bad way to spend your time in retirement.

The longevity hack is doing work you love to do

Nelson Mandela (1918–2013) became the President of South Africa at age 75, whilst the world's richest man, Warren Buffett (b. 1930), still drives to work each day. At 93, Dick Van Dyke (b. 1925) performed an inspirational cameo in *Mary Poppins Returns*, 54 years after starring as Bert in the original *Mary Poppins*. The film also featured Angela Lansbury (b. 1925), whose career across theatre, television and film has spanned a remarkable eight decades.

Working beyond retirement age is not just for the rich and famous though. Nonagenarians like war widow Thelma Zimmerman (b. 1922) continue to live with plenty of purpose and vigour. "I work every Wednesday morning at our church op shop, giving food and clothing to the needy and the homeless," Zimmerman shared with me on *100 Not Out*. Speaking from her home in a South Australian war widows complex, Zimmerman has a full calendar. "I've also been helping clean the church for 25 years. We have a committee meeting once a month on a Tuesday, and then I go to church where I'm on the roster for kitchen duty."

Retirement from professional income-generating work is a logical and desirable step for many people, but retiring from life and no longer contributing to society has disastrous physical, mental and spiritual consequences. Never let age or the word 'retirement' trick you into believing your work is done. If *The Exceptionals* have shown us anything, it's that our work is never done, our value is never diminished; our roles simply change with the passing chapters of life.

Step 5: Enjoy your work or start over

If you've felt that you're too old to change career or create your exceptional life, look no further than 'China's hottest grandpa', Wang Deshun (b. 1936). "People can change their life as many times as they wish,"[16] says Deshun, who today models for Zegna, Reebok and the world's leading fashion designers. After gracing the catwalk at age 79 in 2016, Deshun rose to international stardom, the pin up boy for being able to achieve life's dreams at any age.

"Many say I became an overnight sensation, but I've been preparing for 60 years. At 24 I became a theatre actor, at 44 I started learning English. At 50 years old I went to a gym for the first time. At 70 I was working out regularly. At 79, I went on the runway for the first time," he says. "Today, I am 80 years old and there is still something inside me. I still have dreams to achieve. Our potential can always be explored. When you think that it is too late, be careful. Do not allow this to be an excuse to give up. No one can stop you from succeeding, except yourself."[17]

Just like Wang Deshun – who has also worked as a shoe shiner, a factory worker, and a ticket collector – you are likely to have multiple careers in your life. My history includes working in newsagencies, as a telemarketer, a LEGO® builder and a newspaper delivery boy.

Sometimes the career change can be within the same industry. Matthew McConaughey (b. 1969) studied law before becoming Hollywood's number one romantic comedy actor. After growing stale of the same genre, he refused all rom-com scripts until he landed a role in a drama. Four years after quitting romantic comedies, McConaughey won an Oscar for his portrayal as AIDS patient, Ron Woodroof, in *Dallas Buyers Club*.

If you attempt to find a career that you will do for the rest of your life you're likely to never choose one, as the pressure of that one big decision will render you emotionally paralysed and powerless.

Remember, age is not a barrier. Age is not an excuse. Age is not an alibi. Age is just a number. Your age is a sign of *life*, and life is your blank canvas to create your masterpiece and to write the script of your exceptional life.

> *"Nature determines your age, but you determine your state of mind."*
>
> **– Wang Deshun**

Exceptional Exercise 1.4: What is your life dedicated to?

Let this question nag at you constantly until you can answer it. Giving yourself the time to answer this question is one of your most important tasks in life.

What is *your* life *dedicated* to? Not knowing, or perhaps worse – knowing and *not* dedicating your life to it – will not only suck the life out of you, you'll become bitter and twisted, scourged with resentment, anger, and even hatred. A sad and disconcerting sight is seeing someone with potential who *knows* they are gifted in something and refuses to acknowledge their exceptional nature.

"Our deepest fear is not that we are inadequate," wrote Marianne Williamson in *A Return To Love*. "Our deepest fear is that we are powerful beyond measure. It is our light, not our darkness that most frightens us."[18] What is your *light* that frightens the living daylights out of you? You know, or have a hunch, that you are or could be *crazy good* at something – parenting, turning and fitting, cutting grass, reading contracts, editing, mathematics, astrophysics, negotiating, cooking, running, swimming, gardening, speaking, dancing, singing, designing – yet you shut it off, turn it down and refuse to let it shine.

Denying yourself the greatness and the exceptional life that you deserve benefits no one. In fact, it robs society of a gift.

You can begin the sentence with "my life is dedicated to…" or "the purpose of my life is to…" and then follow it with a verb and an outcome. For me, the purpose of my life is to help humanity rise to exceptional in each area of life and not just one. In my personal life I achieve this through the example I set as a man, husband, father, friend, son, brother, cousin and uncle. In my professional life I do this as a speaker, podcaster, author and mentor.

So, what is *your* life *dedicated* to?

The foundation of your exceptional life is your life purpose

Remember, your life purpose comes *first*, before any other area of life. Your fulfilment during your working hours — whether paid or not — will provide greater longevity than your diet, your exercise habits, your friendship group, your family and your wealth.

Your life purpose is your valued contribution to the world. When the value is gone — when you stop providing value to the world — that's when you begin to really die. Sadly, we can see that in people of *any* age working in jobs they hate — they are dying a slow death, one working day at a time. And not only that, this lack of fulfilment infiltrates most, if not every other area of life.

When you do what you love you wake up with more buzz. You move your body because you know that makes you better at your work; you socialise with great people because those relationships support your life's work; just as your nutrition, your family, your growth and wealth all directly benefit your work. Your spirit is soaked in your work, and the major challenges of life are easier to work through when a strong foundation of fulfilment is derived from your work. If you refuse to live your exceptional life purpose, the odds are you'll die with the painful regret that you didn't summon the courage to live life on your own terms. What outcome do you choose?

▲ ▲ ▲

"Don't hold back. Ten little words.
If it is to be it is up to me."
— Tommy Hafey

How to Do What You Love and Love What You Do *Every Single Day*

When I'm helping people gain clarity on their life purpose, I ask them one question: "Are you doing what you love and loving what you do?" Most of the time the response is blank stares. It's a question that requires elaboration.

Firstly, **what do you love to do**? Your life purpose is dedicated to spending time on activities which you are enthusiastic about. So your answers to this question hold the keys to your future.

Secondly, **what do you do each day**? Write down your daily activities from the time you wake up to the time you go to bed. These answers make up your current reality.

The answer to doing what you love and loving what you do is having similar answers to these two smaller questions. Below is an example from a client of mine, who we'll call Sophie.

> How do you know if you are doing what you love and loving what you do? Draw this table just like Sophie and begin to make gradual progress towards doing more of what you love.

What I love to do	What I did today
Draw	Woke up (checked emails and social media)
Meditate	Made kids breakfast and lunches
Yoga	Did school run
Coffee with friends	Cleaned the house
Travelling	Paid bills and ran errands

Quality family time	School pick up and school activities
Playing tennis	Made dinner, put kids to bed
Interior decorating	Watched TV and checked social media
Reading	Went to bed

Do you think Sophie loves her life right now? It's easy to find the answer when you know how. Is Sophie doing what she loves to do? Is Sophie doing any drawing, meditating, yoga or reading? Is she spending quality time with family, playing tennis or catching up with friends. Based on Sophie's typical day, it's clear she's not doing what she loves.

Sophie's response (and the one I get a lot) is that she doesn't hate her life; she just doesn't love it. She's not unhappy; but she's certainly not happy. This feeling of indifference and numbness is perhaps the truest definition of mediocrity. You can tolerate your existence; you can tolerate mundane daily tasks; but it certainly doesn't feel fulfilling or meaningful.

How to make the columns match up

Firstly, by doing this exercise Sophie now knows what she loves to do and knows that she is *not* doing what she loves to do each day. That clarity is power and for many, enough to shift from a 'can't do' to 'can do' attitude.

Secondly, my recommendation to Sophie is to start small. Begin with 10 or 15 minutes of yoga each day. If you're feeling really adventurous, turn off the TV at night and draw instead, or read your favourite interior design magazines. I know authors who have written a book by committing to as little as one page per day. Progress is better than perfection, and daily progress creates momentum.

After a month, Sophie's typical day looked like this:

What I love to do	What I did today
Draw	Woke up
Meditate	Meditation and yoga
Yoga	Kid's breakfast (ate with them) and did school run (good chats and singing)
Coffee with friends	Coffee with friends
	Errands and bills
Travelling	School pick up and activities
Quality family time	Had dinner together (did gratitudes), helped kids to bed
Playing tennis	Read an interior decorating magazine
Interior decorating	Evening meditation
Reading	Bed

Naturally, Sophie began to feel more fulfilment and sense of purpose in her life rather than feeling stuck in a rinse and repeat cycle of mundane monotony.

What to do if you're still stuck and have no idea what to do with your life

"I don't know what I'm meant to *do* with my life!" It's a statement made by perhaps all of us at some point in our life. And whilst getting clarity on what you love to do is essential, there is a missing piece of the life purpose puzzle that many choose to ignore.

Despite what many will have you believe, your life purpose is more than just what you *do* with your life. On the other side of the coin is your *be*haviour, how you conduct yourself in life, and how you treat others.

Your life achievements will either be tarnished or amplified by who you are as a person. History is littered with individuals who achieved great success but weren't considered very nice human beings. When we leave a job, we rarely remember the work, yet we regularly remember the people – their personalities, how they made us feel, how we related to them, what they did for us and vice versa.

Many workplace cultures have an underlying belief that success is a 'results at all costs' approach, even if that means losing your family relationships, your friendships and your health. Not only is that philosophy incredibly flawed and consequential, it's ignoring the hidden power of the human *being*.

If you're unsure what you want to do with your life right now, you're not alone. Instead of focusing on the doing, decide to put the human *being* into your life purpose. This approach, albeit less tangible for some, has the ability to lay a foundation to your life that your actions and achievements cannot.

▲ ▲ ▲

Put the Human *Being* Into Your Life Purpose

The classic Chinese text the *Tao Te Ching* (written approximately in the 4th century BC) translates to *The Book of the Way and of Virtue*. In this short text (only around 5000 Chinese characters), Lao Tzu outlined the virtues or traits that allow human beings to bring out their most exceptional selves. Those virtues include –

1. Respect
2. Honesty
3. Kindness
4. Helpful

My experience is that when you *behave* more virtuously, the *doing* side of your life purpose manifests far more easily and effortlessly. If you have no idea what you want to *do* in your life, focus instead on how you're *behaving* by measuring yourself in these four virtues. Each day, measure how respectful, honest, kind and helpful you've been. The more you embody these traits, the clearer your life purpose becomes.

You'll find it easier to be respectful, honest, kind and helpful in some activities more than others, and these activities are often what you want to do more of and become the foundation of your life purpose.

Respect

Modern respect differs greatly to its historical counterpart. Respect is best delivered by authentically listening to people. When someone is talking to you, are you checking your phone? Can you look the person in the eye? Can you shut everything out so that all you hear and feel is the other person's words, feelings and emotions? This behaviour applies to your colleagues, your children, your partner, your friends, acquaintances, strangers and most importantly yourself.

Can you see how respect is harder than it sounds? We are so distracted in modern society that being respectful stands out from the crowd. From saying 'please' and 'thank you' at all times, to asking genuine questions (even when you know the answer but you know how much the person loves talking about a subject), you'll find an inner fulfilment arise through the simple act of curiosity. Yes, curiosity breeds respect because when you are curious about another you show that you care and are open to learning. And when you learn, you discover that all people deserve our respect.

Honesty

It has been said before that every lie has a consequence, even the white lies. Even if you tell a lie or withhold the truth in order to *protect* someone, there will be consequences.

Little lies and big lies can have disastrous consequences. Your job in living your exceptional life is to monitor when you lie and work feverishly to develop the courage to tell the often-uncomfortable truth instead.

Do you hold back your true feelings from your partner? Do you soften, rationalise or justify your circumstances? Do you tell people you're "OK" or "fine" when you're really not?

I'm not suggesting you become Jim Carrey in *Liar Liar* and blurt the truth out inappropriately. Instead I urge you to master the art of communication and learn how to tell the truth with vulnerability and compassion for yourself and others. At the same time, avoid taking this message so literally that you remove all fun or humour from your life. I will gleefully lie through my teeth to divert the suspecting recipient (normally my wife or children) away from the scent of my best-laid surprises. Lies have their place in society, just be careful where you place them and be prepared to deal with the consequences they inevitably bring.

> *"No legacy is so rich as honesty."*
> **– William Shakespeare**

Kindness

Eight out of 10 people believe courtesy is a problem in society.[19] From road rage to airport rage, checkout rage to public transport rage, office rage to sports rage, being kind and polite from day to day is exceptional behaviour.

When it's difficult to be kind, it's perhaps more important and exceptional than ever to 'kill them with kindness'. Mindfulness expert and author of *Mindful 2.0*, Vicki Kelly, says the leaders of the next generation will be borne out of the "survival of the kindest". It's easy to be heartless, reckless and unconsciously ruthless today. Do the unpopular – the exceptional – and let your kindness shine when no one expects it.

Helpful

It's interesting that most people who say they do not like their job tend to bring the less-than-best version of themselves to work. You may be an exceptional human being, yet due to the belief about your work, you bring an unhelpful, disrespectful or dishonest version to the office. When you change your inner belief from *I hate my job* to *I look forward to helping my customers or colleagues today* – and you genuinely care to do this, watch your fulfilment soar.

When you behave in this way, you create more clarity on what you do want to *do* with your life. Your life purpose really boils down to who and how you want to help the most. When you're helpful, you're more creative, more confident in your ability and more open to the ideas and opportunities that come your way. And as a bonus, being more helpful will reduce your stress whilst also improving your quality of life.

Exceptional Exercise 1.5: What's your weakness?

All four of these virtues have a degree of overlap. There is likely to be one, though, that stands out as a weakness for you. Would you be wise to be more respectful, honest, kind or helpful? There may be more than one, but for now I suggest focusing on one. Whilst most people are searching for what they're meant to *do* in their life, I encourage you to first ask "who am I here to *be*" and "how can I *be*have more authentically?"

The more you incorporate these four traits into your *behaviour*, the more clear you'll become on what environments organically and effortlessly bring out your respect, honesty, kindness and helpfulness. For me, real life events bring out the best behaviour in me far more easily than the online side of my business. Speaking from the stage, engaging with human beings in the flesh, and having long-form discussions are far better for me than online webinars, emails and social media.

It took me three years of my business life to realise this and structure my business to align with my personality and virtues, and even though that may seem a long time, I'm so thankful I worked it out in three years and not 33 years! No matter how long it takes you to unleash your exceptional *be*haviour, the fulfilment you receive from living virtuously in accordance with your life purpose creates an indestructible foundation on which to live your exceptional life.

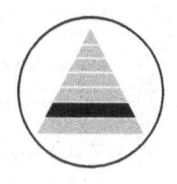

MOVEMENT

"To live longer; move more."
- Dr Walter Bortz

Welcome to perhaps the most underrated and misunderstood ingredient for living an exceptional life. Whilst most people are feeling guilty or making excuses for not exercising, the longest-lived people around the world are actually...not exercising.

For the *Exceptionals* who are exercising – the 70, 80 and 90-year-old world record holders and Mary, your overactive mid-week tennis-playing, garden-loving next door neighbour whose kids just wish "Mum would slow down" – they are moving in ways they love to move, rather than exercising because they 'should'. They're dancing, swimming, running, playing football, doing yoga, tai chi, horse-riding, cycling, lifting weights, surfing, and so on because they love to, not because they have to. For *The Exceptionals*, movement is a lifestyle choice. For everyone else, movement is a lifestyle chore.

The truth is that less than 20% of the population is sufficiently physically active, and it's causing havoc around the planet. It's even suggested that more than 40% of all dementia would disappear if we moved regularly, and many cancers, diabetes and heart disease all list a lack of movement as a major risk factor.

So what does it take to become an *Exceptional*? Firstly, if 'exercise' feels like a dirty word, replacing it with 'movement' is key. Secondly, know that moving your body becomes more important the older you get. And finally, moving regularly in ways that you love may go a long way to preventing an undignified death.

Enjoy the modern world of technology and at the same time prioritise the time-honoured movements such as gardening or going for a walk to get some fresh air. Exercise because you love to, not because your friend has lost more weight than you.

To ascend from mediocre to magnificent movement, the responsibility is yours and yours alone, and thankfully there are inspirational mentors to help you make it happen. It gives me great pleasure to introduce you to the world of the exceptional movers and shakers.

Transform from Exercise to Movement

"People were so excited, I couldn't get out the front door." An 84-year-old nun was sharing with me how she had become a celebrity in the triathlon world and now everyone wanted a piece of her. "I'm thinking, 'what about the professionals?' They are working their butts off and they aren't getting the publicity they deserve. They deserve the pictures on the front page every day. Instead it's me, this little old lady getting all of the attention."

This little old lady was Sister Madonna Buder, a Roman Catholic nun from Spokane, Washington. Buder had just become the oldest woman in history to complete an Ironman Triathlon when she crossed the line at the 2012 Ironman Canada in under 17 hours. Her rise to fame included becoming a Nike ambassador with her very own television advertisement and being inducted into the USA Triathlon Hall of Fame.

Jan Smith (b. 1944) became the oldest Australian woman to scale Mount Everest when she reached the summit the day after her 68th birthday. The Melbourne grandmother and psychologist started mountaineering when she was 65 and has scaled six of the *Seven Peaks* – the seven highest mountains in the seven continents on the planet.

Accountant Don Riddington (b. 1944), who began swimming when he was 50, became the oldest Australian to cross the English Channel when he conquered the treacherous route at age 68 in 2013.

Nonagenarian Heather Lee (b. 1927) is the world's fastest walker in her age group. Medical doctor Walter Bortz (b. 1930) has completed over 40 marathons. He celebrated his 80th birthday by running the Boston Marathon in 2010. Jack LaLanne (1914–2011), a self-confessed childhood "sugarholic", became host of the first health and fitness television program *The Jack LaLanne Show*. On his 70th birthday he swam for one mile tied to 70 boats.

You're never too old to do anything. Whatever excuses you or others have, there are countless *Exceptionals* who have done what society says cannot or should not be done. Not one *Exceptional* has ever bought into the belief of being too old. Whilst their legs may not be as fast, their mind remains more willing than ever. *The Exceptionals* do not need to be shaken out of bed to go exercise. It isn't a grind. They exercise because they *love* to. For *The Exceptionals*, exercise is not a lifestyle chore; it's a lifestyle choice.

Exercise has been a public health failure

The aforementioned *Exceptionals* who excel at exercise – training for mountaineering, triathlons, sprints and competition – are in the small percentage of people who love to exercise or get enough of it. "Exercise has been an unmitigated public health failure," according to Blue Zones founder, Dan Buettner. "Fewer than 18% of people in the developed world exercise enough. So, it isn't working for the vast majority," Buettner told Jay Shetty's *On Purpose* podcast.[1] "As we see obesity on the rise in most countries, school kids aren't moving enough. It's (exercise) just not been a successful strategy to deal with our health care problems. It sells a lot of books, it sells gym memberships and gadgets and TV shows and yoga classes. It's a great business, but it's not doing the job, and I feel like the *Emperor's New Clothes* (saying this) – by pointing out (that) it ain't working!

"People think they have to pump iron, run triathlons and break a sweat, but actually walking gives you about 90% of the physical activity of training for a marathon. If you're 80 years old and you can walk a mile (1.6km) in under 17 minutes it adds about six years to your life expectancy. Just the act of walking!"[2]

How much constant and mindless movement do you have in your daily life? Can you – and do you – walk one mile in under 17 minutes on a regular basis? Are you outsourcing a lot of your mindless movement to cleaners, gardeners or using your car or public transport more than you could? Are you succumbing to modern conveniences that easily and unconsciously reduce your daily movement? I'm not suggesting you have to clean your entire house, do all the gardening and sell your car. Instead, consider if you've lost the balance between modern conveniences and incidental movement.

Longevity cultures don't exercise

If the thought of daily exercise has you shuddering, the good news is you don't need to be an exercise junkie to join *The Exceptionals*. "In Blue Zones, people don't exercise – at least not in the way that we think of exercise," Buettner continues. "In Blue Zones, people are getting plenty of physical activity into their 90s and 100s because they live in environments that nudge them mindlessly into moving every 20 minutes or so. Every time they go to work, every time they go to a friend's house, every time they go out to eat is an occasion to walk. They don't have a button to push for the housework and kitchen work – they do it by hand. They have gardens out the back. They're in constant, mindless movement which is what I believe we need to start thinking about if we're going to make healthier cities."[3]

On the Japanese island of Okinawa, movement comes from their traditional lifestyle. All Okinawans have a garden they tend to, they eat sitting on the floor – which means they get up and down many times each day – and do a lot of walking. None of it is structured exercise. The Greek island of Ikaria has no gyms or state of the art yoga studios. Instead, they walk and hike the undulating island, swim and body surf in the ocean, dance at their festivals, and tend their land.

In California, the graceful agers of Seventh Day Adventist community Loma Linda are partial to regular exercise, and they also have lifestyle and religious rituals that encourage regular movement. During the Sabbath, Loma Lindans are likely to hike or walk with family and friends on the day of rest and worship. On the Italian island of Sardinia, men living the traditional shepherd lifestyle walk on average eight kilometres per day whilst the women are physically active around the home.[4]

Move like Giannis and Joanna

Each year when I host the 100 Not Out Longevity Experience in Ikaria, we stay in the village of Nas at Thea's Inn and Restaurant. Our host, Thea Parikos (b. 1962), has an auntie and uncle, Joanna (b. 1935) and Giannis Meli (b. 1932), who live half way up the hill, overlooking the Aegean Sea and almost every other house in the community. To come into the commercial hub of Nas (a single street mind you), Joanna has to walk down approximately 60 uneven, somewhat deep steps. She does this with great speed and agility, undoubtedly to the concern of some of her neighbours. Giannis, despite slowing down gradually each year, still maintains the alacrity to navigate these steps with confidence.

If either Giannis or Joanna want to visit neighbours or go to the village to dine out, buy some coffee or flour (they are self-sufficient for everything else), they must walk down – and back up – the steps. This mindless movement, built in to the Ikarian lifestyle, is what many of us are missing. We have to consciously *nudge* ourselves at first into mindless movement, and then make it permanent. Cook from scratch instead of zapping pre-prepared meals, use a basket or bags instead of using a trolley, park your car further away so you need to walk more, and take the option of walking or riding instead of driving. In many ways, the answer is to be *less* efficient in order to be *more* effective. If the thought of all that extra *time* moving mindlessly makes you uncomfortable, combine it with listening to podcasts or audiobooks, calling your loved ones or conducting walking meetings.

Movement is more important than diet for a long life

"Another gold medal for Australia!" Ruth Frith (1909–2014) had just won one of her six gold medals in athletics at the 2009 World Masters Games in Sydney. Sitting down to do an interview with the ABC shortly after, Frith was asked about her workout routine.

"Monday I do weights, pushups, ride the bike and do some stretching. Tuesday I do that again; Wednesday I do practical training on the field. Thursday I do the same again and Friday I do weights again." Asked if she thought she had an advantage over her competitors because of her workout regime, Frith replied: "Well when I'm with them I find out they don't do anything. A lot of them don't even train!"[5]

When asked her recommendations for movement, Frith insisted: "Even if you only do three days a week. You must, you can't expect to keep going forever doing what you did. I started (athletics) when I was 74. What I did when I was 74 you can't do when your 84."[6]

Frith wasn't lying; she really did begin her Masters athletics career at 74. Her daughter, Helen Searle, is a Commonwealth Games silver medallist and represented Australia at the 1960 and 1964 Olympic Games, and continued on into Masters athletics when her professional career ended. For years, Frith would go along and mind the bags of Helen and her fellow club members until one day she had her epiphany, as she told me on *100 Not Out*: "Enough of the bag minding, it's my turn to give this a go!"

Frith, who lived to 104, was so exceptional that she won some of her gold medals purely because she was the only competitor in her age group, and she still holds some of the 25 world records she set. Like many centenarians, Frith was regularly asked the perennial question, "What's your secret?" to which she replied, "It's not diet, because I don't eat vegetables. So it doesn't have anything to do with the diet!"[7]

Frith's comments can come across as flippant and some health professionals might be squirming at the idea that movement trumps diet for healthy longevity. However, anecdotal evidence suggests that whilst a great diet is wonderful for improving quality of life and can be a great healing aid, it doesn't contribute to longevity in the same way movement does.

Countless *Exceptionals* have shared with me their daily diet on *100 Not Out*. Lavinia Petrie (b. 1943) runs 10km in 40 minutes on her way to gold medals for Australia. She celebrates with a "hamburger with the lot" and a trip to the bakery.

Sister Madonna Buder is partial to a pastry, whilst octogenarian Ruth Heidrich (b. 1938) is a vegan athlete who's run over 60 marathons and multiple triathlons. Alan and Janette Murray ran 366 marathons in 366 days in barefoot runners eating nothing but raw fruits and vegetables.

Longevity cultures all have a wholefood-based diet with considerable differences. The Okinawans thrive on rice and fish and consume very few fruits, whereas the Loma Lindans are largely vegetarian or vegan.[8] Corn is the staple of Nicoya, Costa Rica (the South American Blue Zone), whilst the Greek Blue Zone of Ikaria enjoys a Mediterranean diet that differs to the Sardinian version.[9] And of course, Australian Ruth Frith didn't eat vegetables! If you're looking for anything in common food-wise, Blue Zones founder Dan Buettner says the only food all longevity cultures have in common is the consumption of beans. While *The Exceptionals* may not share the same diet, they all have a love of moving their bodies.

There is no supplement for exercise

From now on in this book, whenever you see the word exercise, I want you to think of movement, particularly if you have felt an aversion to structured exercise.

One of the medical profession's biggest champions of healthy ageing is geriatrician Dr Walter Bortz. A doctor who more than walks his talk, Bortz is a prolific author on graceful ageing, including *We Live Too Short and Die Too Long*, *Dare To Be 100* and *Getting Older For Dummies*.

Bortz's own exceptional life was shaped by the death of his father when Bortz was 39. "My father was my Alpha and Omega figure," Bortz told me in 2013. "When he died I was just bereft. I couldn't sleep, work, or think. I was a son who had just lost his dad. I rescued myself with three things: I started to run – and I'm about to run my 43rd consecutive annual marathon. Second, we moved to California, and third, I became a geriatrician. All of those were balm for my injured soul."

Bortz, who describes movement as "the best anti-depressant there is" is widely known for his commitment to his own movement but also to movement as a healer. "There is no supplement for exercise. The right dietary advice is to be active. It's a lot cheaper to be healthy than it is to be sick."

Bortz has so much faith in the power of fitness that he calls it a "30 year age offset. A fit person of 80 is an unfit person of 50". In addition, if you've been inspired by the stories of late starters including Madonna Buder, Jan Smith and Don Riddington, Bortz even has his own law for transforming in later years: "Bortz law says 'never too late to start; always too soon to stop.' How you age is negotiable. It's up to you, not up to anyone else."

Are your excuses lies?

So why do less than 20% of the population exercise regularly? One answer is time, or people's perceived lack of time. The negative mantra of most of us is: "I don't have time to exercise." The truth is any excuse is a lie. 'I don't have time' is just another way of saying *I have other responsibilities or tasks that I consider more important* such as sleeping, getting the kids ready for school, working, resting, catching up with friends or watching TV. Excuses overtly demonstrate what our true values are, which we'll explore in the section on family.

Excuses are far more inclined to arise around exercise and less so around movement. Many people find it easier to go for a walk along the beach than they do going for a run. Your job in living your exceptional life is to find ways you love to move your body – it could be walking or hiking, dancing or swimming, water polo, roller skating, skateboarding, horse-riding or any other type of physical activity you do for pure enjoyment.

Your biggest challenge will be drowning out the noise of *excusitis* that dribbles out of our mouths so unconsciously that a learned helplessness in this area of life is created. Many of us feel like we're so busy doing everything yet not winning at anything. We feel mediocre at almost everything we do. Our job is OK, our health is OK, our relationships are OK, our finances are OK; our life is just OK. Nothing is exceptional, because we feel we don't have the time to make anything magnificent – and there's no pressure to rise to exceptional when average is socially accepted.

Resist movement at your own peril

Your job and responsibility in living your exceptional life is to believe in your own divinity, as difficult as that may be. That doesn't mean you don't have challenges, down times, frustrations or setbacks. That's equally a part of living an exceptional life. What sets *The Exceptionals* apart, whether it be in movement or any part of life, is the standards they have. Most people look at the standards set by *Exceptionals* and think they're either unachievable or unreasonable, and for them, they may be. But for you, the *Exceptional*, you have a standard which can not only be reached, achieved and sustained, but when you go below that standard, you are quick to respond, knowing that your identity as an *Exceptional* is so hardwired into your heart and soul that you refuse to live below your standards for long at all.

Often the most powerful way to create change is to confront and visualise the physical changes resulting from years of ignoring movement. Do you have a friend that was incredibly attractive or handsome in their teenage years, 20s and perhaps 30s, who 'let themselves go' when they either finished school, fell in love, started working longer hours, or had children? What changed for them? What happened is their values changed. Children became more important than movement. Work became more important than friends, and sleeping in with your partner became more important than a morning workout. None of these examples are bad or wrong. Instead, they each bring with them a consequence.

All of those examples are ones from my own life. Where the trap of mediocrity lives is *how long* you live in those changes for. Yes, there are times when you must work extra long hours, but when do you pull the trigger and arrest control of your own calendar and personal health regime? Most people will never reclaim their power back. They now give their time and energy away to their work, their children, their TV and very little to their own selves. They live according to everyone else's demands and values and are on the path to living with regret.

If I'm coming down hard here, it's because for some reason, the resistance to exceptional movement is often more hardwired than changing your life's purpose, reinvigorating your marriage or reconnecting with your estranged family or friends. And my concern for you or anyone who denies the value of movement for an exceptional life, is that you are potentially on the fast-track to an undignified end.

▲ ▲ ▲

The Mediocre Movement Disaster

Picture this – you're sitting alone in a small room, reclined in a lounge chair, staring at a wall with a single picture frame hanging from it. It's a three-generation family photo – you, your soul mate, your children and your grandchildren. The photo was taken just over nine years ago at your 73rd birthday. Up until then, you lived a fabulous life. You prioritised a family who loves you, did work that you love to do, ate well, created some magical memories both at home and abroad, and had accumulated a handsome nest egg that meant you would never need to think about money again. Or so you thought.

Shortly after your 73rd birthday, life took the sharpest of U-turns. Slowly but surely, you began to notice a decline in your ability to think clearly, remember short-term details, and recall people's names. Whilst you attempted to minimise it and fob it off, it became clear that something was seriously amiss when one spring morning you went down the street to pick up some bread and didn't know how to get home. Sitting in the car, trembling, shaking and screaming, the realisation that dementia was about to strangle your life had just taken hold. You were in the throes of cognitive decline and your entire life was about to go into shutdown.

Amidst your panic attack existed a disturbing clarity of thought that was equally confronting: what would become of your relationship with your spouse, children and grandchildren? What about your regular coffee dates with lifelong friends, the promise of future international travel and the magic moments with loved ones? Your entire quality of life as you knew it was under threat; not just the big things, but if you couldn't find your way home from the bakery, how would you complete the small tasks of daily life? All your dreams, both big and small, disappeared with the resulting diagnosis of dementia, and the very heart of your life was swiftly ripped out when you were moved out of home to a care facility.

After a couple of years, the physical, mental, and emotional stress became too much for your spouse. Now, only sorrow lived in the eyes of your soul mate. Yes, you had lived a great life together, but now your partner's only thought was of the future and how different it could have, and was supposed to have been.

Your children have tried desperately to remember you as the parent pre-dementia, yet the longer you live, the harder it is, as the fortnightly visits with the grandchildren became more and more heart-wrenching in proportion to your decline. It's clear your younger grandchildren will never really know who you really were. They remember you as the grandparent who asked the same two questions over and over again, and randomly became incoherent or frantic. Your friends no longer visit; they prefer to hold on to the memories of when you were a functioning member of society.

And sadly, what you will never be fully aware of is the financial disaster your dementia has served the family. Your financial legacy has been sacrificed in exchange for keeping you as comfortable as possible for as long as possible. The deposits you intended to finance for your children's family homes, the school-fee help you intended to leave behind and the financial security your partner would live with are now gone. The pension beckons for your spouse, confined to the time-rich cash-poor elderly community caused by the slow, drawn-out death of a partner. More than 40 years of hard work to accumulate financial security has been blown to smithereens in under a decade.

As you sit reclined in that lounge chair and begin to take your final breaths, the peace that you wish you would die with is instead clouded with regret that you failed to place a vital piece in the puzzle of an exceptional life. And sadly, you're not alone.

Dementia is the worst way to die

The above example, with the details clearly differing for each person, is reality for approximately 50 million people *right now* with 10 *million* new diagnoses being made each year. By the year 2030 there will be 82 million people with dementia and by 2050 that number will be almost double, reaching 152 million people.[10]

And whilst dementia is more common amongst older people, it is *not* a normal part of the ageing process (in which case we would all get it, just like losing our teeth at childhood is a normal part of the ageing process). Whatever age you are right now you are either creating or preventing the seeds of dementia from growing. In fact, dementia takes between 20 and 50 years to develop before a diagnosis can be made, so even if you're in your 20s or 30s this section is important.[11] The decisions you make at this stage of your life have the power to set the tone for brain health for many years to come.

If you don't fancy spending the last 3000 days of your life confined to a dementia ward in a high-care nursing home, you're not alone. When I'm presenting and I ask people what they believe the worst way to die is, the overwhelming response is dementia (there's always someone that says being burnt alive).

Dementia impacts the family of the patient more than any other disease. It takes four people to look after one patient, and due to the cognitive decline, it has far greater emotional impact on the family. The person they *knew* for so long slowly becomes someone who doesn't know anyone around them, which is heartbreaking for everyone involved.

Adding insult to injury is the diagnosis to death time. Whilst the average is around 4.5 years, dementia can be more than a dozen years for some, with people diagnosed before 70 living for a decade longer than their older counterparts.[12]

Longevity is the cause of dementia

The scary, and equally mostly wonderful thing about our modern world is how quickly we have increased our life expectancy (the average age of death across a population). Since 1900, global life expectancy has more than doubled from between 30 and 40 years of age and is now above 70 years. Given how slow evolution tends to be, this development in only five generations is quite extraordinary. The World Health Organization has Japan atop the life expectancy ladder at 83.7 (both sexes), followed by Switzerland, Singapore and Australia (82.8). The UK is 20th with 81.2, the USA is 38th with 77.8 while Sierra Leone brings in the tail at 50.1.[13]

Life expectancy by country

Rank	Country	Male	Female	Both	Health Adjusted
1	Japan	80.5	86.8	83.7	74.9
2	Switzerland	81.3	85.3	83.4	73.1
3	Singapore	80.0	86.1	83.1	73.9
4	Australia	80.9	84.8	82.8	71.9
20	United Kingdom	79.4	83.0	81.2	71.4
38	United States	74.7	81.1	77.8	68.1
183	Sierra Leone	49.3	50.8	50.1	44.4

Source: World Health Organization (2015)

Given such rapid change in a small amount of time, dementia is regarded as a somewhat modern phenomenon. "We do know that 150 years ago not many people reached 70 so it (dementia) was regarded as a bit of a rarity," says Professor Michael Woodward, head of Aged Care at Melbourne hospital Austin Health. "Now, with the life expectancy over 80 for males and females, it's (dementia) becoming very common. So really we have (so many more cases of) dementia because we're living longer."

Given we've only been dealing with this exceptional longevity for two generations, we still have so much to learn about the art of ageing well, let alone dementia. Many of us are unsure *how* to age well because we haven't necessarily had the parents or grandparents living long enough to show us. And similarly, just like social security benefits weren't a burden on society when life expectancy was 65, dementia and aged care wasn't a burden until we all started living longer.

Longevity therefore is nothing to hang your hat on if your final chapter is undignified, lonely, dependent and downright depressing. Whilst Australia sits fourth on the longevity ladder, she plummets to 15th for *quality* of life. Statistically speaking, the last 11 years of life in the 'lucky country' are spent in a state of disease.

To many in society, these are just numbers. Statistics mean very little to us until we become one of them. Personally, spending the last 11 years in poor health is one of my worst nightmares.

This is not a problem that will go away, nor will it get any smaller. Our job as *Exceptionals* is to ensure we avoid buying into the belief that dementia is a normal part of ageing and to live the principles of the *Exceptionals* that have been proven to prevent dementia.

So what exactly is dementia?

Dementia itself is not technically a disease, but a syndrome. It is an overall term for diseases and conditions characterised by declining memory, language, problem-solving and other thinking skills. Alzheimer's disease is the most common form of dementia, making up between 60 and 70% of all cases around the world. Others include Lewy Body disease, vascular as well as frontotemperal dementia.

Dementia is now the most common cause of death amongst women over 80. It is the third leading cause of death (behind heart disease and stroke) in high-income countries. Deaths due to dementia more than doubled between 2000 and 2016, making it the fifth leading cause of death in 2016 (compared to 14th in 2000).[14]

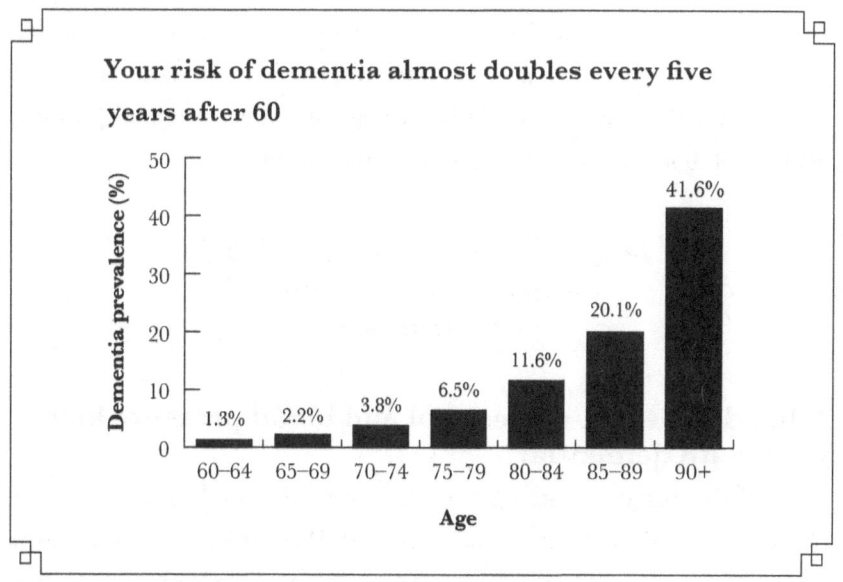

Your risk of dementia almost doubles every five years after 60

Age	Dementia prevalence (%)
60–64	1.3%
65–69	2.2%
70–74	3.8%
75–79	6.5%
80–84	11.6%
85–89	20.1%
90+	41.6%

Source: World Health Organization (2012)

Prevent dementia by 42%

Amid all the dementia doom and gloom, as always there is another side to the coin. If you're as determined as I am to have a more graceful and dignified death than dementia, you'll be happy to know a pathway exists that puts the odds in your favour. If you think back to the dementia example I gave at the beginning of this chapter, you may have noticed that the lifestyle ingredient I purposely left out was movement.

"We know that we can probably prevent 42% of all dementia if everybody in society was sufficiently physically active. That's a pretty powerful intervention." That's a pretty powerful statement from one of the planet's must trusted and respected voices in geriatrics – Professor Michael Woodward.

When Professor Woodward shared this with me on *100 Not Out*, he explained that being "sufficiently physically active" means 30 minutes per day. Of the 48 half-hour segments we have available to us each day, all we need to do is dedicate just *one* of them to movement.

Unfortunately most people are unaware how severe the consequences of removing movement from their lifestyle truly is. Whilst we recognise fatigue, being sluggish and unfit as short-term effects of poor movement, the real impact goes much deeper, all the way to the brain. Poor movement habits have also been shown to impact quality of sleep, blood pressure, cholesterol, bone density, obesity, cancer and diabetes.

> *"Being fit is armour. It protects you from all types of indignities, including Alzheimer's."*
> *– Dr Walter Bortz*

What do obesity, cholesterol and blood pressure have to do with dementia?

One of the biggest mistruths or misconceptions in health is that all chronic diseases are separate and unrelated. We think our blood pressure has nothing to do with our cholesterol, and that diabetes has nothing to do with dementia. We think an autoimmune condition is not related to cancer, and that a skin condition is unrelated to stress. We grow up singing, "the hip bone's connected to the leg bone", yet we somehow forget this truth when it comes to the organs and systems within the body.

Dr. Miia Kivipelto of the Karolinska Institute in Sweden led a 21-year study on 1449 individuals that found people who were obese in middle age were twice as likely to develop dementia when they got old as those who were of normal weight.[15] For those who also had high cholesterol and high blood pressure in middle age, the risk of dementia was *six* times higher.[16] Could these common health conditions be warning signs of what's to come? Of course! Do we listen to our body when it whispers to us in the form of high blood pressure or high cholesterol (conditions which we don't *feel* like a broken bone or sore back)? Absolutely not. We instead take a medication and carry on with life as usual (43 and 58 million Americans take statins and blood pressure medication, respectively), making little to no adjustments to our life, unconsciously writing the script for an undignified final decade of life.

Prevent dementia by multi-tasking

But what if by transforming from mediocre to exceptional movement, we not only massively reduced our risk of dementia, but also our risk for heart disease, stroke, cancer, diabetes and many other chronic diseases? And on top of that we enjoyed improved concentration, energy levels, daily resilience, sleep quality, libido, moods and more?

"It's fortuitous that the very same lifestyle changes that you need to do to keep your heart healthy are generally the lifestyle changes that will also keep your brain healthy," explains Professor Woodward. "Isn't it wonderful that we can multi-task? We can be trying to change people's attitude to health for one purpose but it might also have benefits in other areas. Let's face it, it's far better in terms of your own self-esteem and your interactions with your peers, to be regularly exercising and fit than not. So there are immediate benefits from these lifestyle changes. It's not just an investment in your future 30 or 40 years down the track.

"It's a worrying thing however that we are getting increased numbers of people with obesity and diabetes and I think that's where a lot of attention needs to be. These are risk factors, not just for heart disease, not just for cancer but also for Alzheimer's disease. We can also reduce our risk of Alzheimer's if we keep our brain active (and) if we keep socially engaged."

As Professor Woodward explains, preventing cognitive decline is not as simple as moving well. Your social life and sense of purpose is incredibly important. So is your family history. There is not one cure-all for dementia, and even the most socially and physically active people have developed cognitive decline. Importantly, if you or someone you love are showing signs of dementia, nothing could be more urgent than getting informed and taking proactive steps to stop the decline and potentially improve symptoms. See the Endnotes section for further reading so that you can become informed and empowered on exceptional brain health.

Take Responsibility for Your Vitality

Ten little words were the mantra of Australian rules football icon, Tommy Hafey (1931–2014). His fierce determination to take responsibility for all areas of his life is what made Hafey truly exceptional. Hafey's habits as a footballer and coach followed him his entire life. Without exception, Hafey would wake up at 5:20 each weekday morning and would set out on a 5km run. He would then complete 251 push-ups and go for a swim in Melbourne's Port Phillip Bay.

On returning home he would complete 700 sit-ups, before enjoying breakfast with his wife Maureen. He once made a New Year's Resolution to his children that he would not eat lollies, biscuits or cake. That lasted for 42 years right up until his death from melanoma.

Hafey's commitment to his health became a talking point for many Australians: "A lot of people do ask me, 'I don't want to be rude but how old are you?' and I think, 'Well I'd never thought anything of it because I've never stopped doing the work that I do'.[17]

"(My belief is that) you put your head down and give it everything you've got. If you don't make it, that's not failure. Not having a go is failure. Commit yourself and don't be thinking 'dammit I wish I could have it all over again because I didn't give it my best shot'. Ten little words – 'If it is to be it is up to me' – and I want you to put a big circle around the word 'me' because that's where it all comes back to – it's you."[18]

These words are taken from an advertisement Hafey featured in for Jeep automobiles to celebrate its 70th anniversary in 2011. The incredible thing is that Hafey, the ambassador and personification of Jeep's message of *Don't Hold Back* was 79 years old at the time.

Hafey's life came to a quick and unexpected end, dying within a matter of weeks from advanced melanoma, 24 years after having a melanoma cut from his back. Despite the speed at which cancer killed him, Hafey was still 82 when he died, and had lived an incredible quality of life for all but the final three months – a duration most would gratefully accept in preference to the more than 10 years many suffer for.

Love your movement and enjoy your exercise

"I cannot do indoor exercise and enjoy it," Madonna Buder emphasised to me. "My enjoyment is to be out in nature in what God created. Sitting on a bike inside watching the numbers turn around makes me feel like a lab rat and I lose my spirit, because that's not the way we are constructed. We are constructed with mind, body and soul and when one of the three gets out of balance then we're in for trouble.

"I've noticed that in myself – when I get so obsessed with trying to get in X number of miles – then I'm driving myself into burnout and then I've lost the urge to do it because it's robbed me of the thrill of being free."

When you do as Buder does and move in ways that make you feel free, you can rest assured you're moving exceptionally. For me, riding a bike, going for a walk or a hike bring about great feelings of freedom. For others, it's surfing, and for others it's running, dancing, rock climbing, kiteboarding or some form of sport. We all feel free moving in different ways. When your movement becomes your exercise and your exercise becomes your movement it will be a lifestyle choice rather than a chore.

Slow down at your own risk

Bill Stevens (b. 1928) is an aqua aerobics and Body Pump instructor at Melbourne YMCA leisure centres and is described by his clients as "unique" and "one of a kind". Bill is over 90 years of age and at one stage taught 35 classes per week. "Now I'm down to 12 and I fill in for a few," the exceptional nonagenarian shared with me on *100 Not Out*.

"My kids tell me to slow down but I have no problems. Four weeks ago I broke a rib doing one of my classes. That was pretty painful but you get on with it. I went overseas last year and I showed my passport at passport control. The lady looked at me – and 'fitness instructor' is on my departure card – and she said, 'You're a fitness instructor, still working?' I said 'yeah'."

Stevens, who spent more than 40 years working as a wine executive, walks his talk by participating regularly in group classes at the gym and running five kilometres every couple of days. He's been a pescetarian (fish-eating vegetarian) for the last 25 years and enjoys two glasses of wine with dinner each night.

"I don't feel more than 50. I've never been old so I don't know what it feels like being old," he says. "If I had a plan, my plan would be to do this until the day I die. If I die on the job one day, doing what I love, then so be it."

If you tell your parents to slow down or have children telling you to take it easy, keep Bill Stevens and his fellow *Exceptionals* in your thoughts. Only 9% of men and 6% of women who are 75 or older get enough physical activity.[19] To be a truly exceptional mover one has to be more than the odd one out. If anyone ever tells you to slow down, let it only be because they're unable to keep up with you.

Take a leaf out of the book of Stevens, Buder, Riddington, Smith and the aforementioned *Exceptionals*. You don't have to be a fast runner, climb Mount Everest or be the Iron Nun. All you need to do is lead by example, which you are already doing. The only question you need to ask is whether you are fulfilled by the example you set. If your movement habits are mediocre, what impact is that having on yourself and the people around you, and are you prepared to experience their consequences?

> *"We don't need to slow down; we need to calm down."*
> *– Bob Proctor*

Know the difference between health and fitness

It's easy to think being fit is the same as being healthy. I was first made aware of this significant distinction by world-renowned sports coach, chiropractor and complementary medicine doctor, Dr Phillip Maffetone. According to Maffetone, "Fitness is the ability to perform physical activity. Health is the ideal balance of all the systems of the body – the nervous, muscular, skeletal, circulatory, digestive, lymphatic, and hormonal."[20]

In other words, just because you can run 100 metres in 10 seconds, lift heavy weights or ride a bike for 100km doesn't make you healthy. It makes you fit. If you never fully understand the difference between health and fitness, you're unlikely to ever truly embrace the purpose of magnificent movement. Instead, you'll be measuring yourself against the clock or weight rack (fitness) instead of listening to your body and the feedback it's giving you (health).

For some reason many people are determined to 'push through' when they are exercising, believing that 'no pain no gain' is the only measure of success. For elite athletes this may be the case on rare occasions, but even for them, this philosophy is not the cornerstone of success. The attainment of health first, followed then by the pursuit of fitness, is the *exceptional* order. For everyone else, looking good on the outside trumps functioning well on the inside, until it's too late.

I learnt the hard way

Our first child, Maya, was born on January 1, 2010. Shortly after her birth I decided I would complete my first half ironman triathlon in November. Amongst family time and keeping our business running, I began training for the 1.9km swim, 90km bike ride and 21.1km run. Saturday and Sunday mornings were long rides followed by long runs. Weekday mornings and lunch breaks were spent swimming and running, and as a result of the training load, I was tired when I was at home with the family and just wanted to rest.

At a time when life was meant to somewhat simplify (work, sleep, eat and change nappies), life had become unnecessarily complicated. Not only was I tired at home, I was late to most of my training sessions and was cutting it fine with my workload as well. In short, I was over-committed and I refused to do anything about it or heed the warning signs. On a drizzly Melbourne Cup Day, just two weeks before my half ironman debut, I was on a training ride when a car at an intersection didn't see me coming. It crossed the intersection safely however I was forced to brake, skidded and fell into a gutter, shattering and dislocating my left shoulder.

My over-committed life was bound to reach a breaking point, and this was it. Amidst the turbulence of becoming a father, supporting Sarah, Maya and our business, I had not only committed to bite off more than I could chew, I had now paid a hefty price for my commitment to being too exceptional. Frustratingly, I had also passed those consequences on to Sarah, Maya and our extended family, who nursed me through two surgeries and the resulting rehabilitation.

In hindsight the stupidity of it all is ridiculous. But sometimes we are blinded in the moment. Even Dr Walter Bortz, who had to stop running at 88 after completing 45 marathons, acknowledged that he put too much focus on exercise. "The Greeks said, 'Everything in moderation' and I was not moderate. I think I just wore (my legs) out, just gone from too much use," Bortz said in an interview in 2018. "I never had any distinction as a runner – I was once interviewed by PBS for coming in last in the Boston Marathon – but I love to run. I'm terribly upset when I see runners running and I can't do it. It bothers me."[21]

Getting the balance right with your exceptional movement is vital. It may take years to discover it, and it may also change overnight. Personally, I completely missed the memo telling me to slow down when Maya was born, instead ramping it up when the opposite was in order. Movement shouldn't be something you're stressing about fitting in. It's akin to worrying you'll be late for a meditation or yoga class; it defeats the purpose.

Unless you're a professional athlete or high-level amateur with a magnificent obsession for competition, your movement shouldn't feel like another appointment you need to get to. Instead, movement is a way of life, a lifestyle choice that can last for hours or just minutes; the type of experience you're grateful to have the privilege to be able to do. Exceptional movement will give you a quality of life nothing else can, and contribute to your longevity more than any other health practice.

> *"If you can only do one thing for your health, remain physically active. Being active is the life-saver."*
> **– Stephen Jepson**

SOCIAL LIFE

*"Everyone wants to ride with you in the limo.
But what you want is someone who will take
the bus with you when the limo breaks down."
– Oprah Winfrey*

Socialise or die an undignified death. Nothing could be more stark when it comes to the example set by *The Exceptionals*. Whether you're an introvert or a raging extrovert, human connection is life-saving, life-extending and life-enriching.

Whilst many of us declare "I don't have time to socialise," *The Exceptionals* know that time is all we have, and engaging with humanity is an investment in the present *and* the future.

The Exceptionals recognise that the perfect diet, exceptional wealth or the best meditation practice doesn't come close to the life-extending power of socialising. Research now proves that an exceptional social life is more important for longevity than the perfect diet.[1]

The Exceptionals love where they live and embrace community for its original Latin meaning of *public spirit*. And whilst *The Exceptionals* may be patriotic, their personal culture – their peer group, beliefs and values – far outweighs national culture. You become who you hang around, and nothing can be more powerful (or difficult) than improving your peer group.

Your family doesn't come first in the recipe for longevity. Any centenarian Holocaust survivor who lost every member of their family will prove that. An exceptional peer group supports you through the tough times and contributes more to your quantity of life than your family. For many *Exceptionals*, their friends are their family and their family are their friends.

An exceptional social life is a superfood of longevity that science is yet to really understand. Science *knows* that human connection heals, enriches and extends life, but doesn't know how or why. No medical specialist will ever be able to stick a needle in your arm and get a reading on your social life. May this chapter act as that needle, and may the stories of *The Exceptionals* provide you with the nutrients to transform and enrich your connection to humanity.

⬥ ⬥ ⬥

The Exceptional Social Life Prototype

In 1900, heart disease was an uncommon cause of death. By the 1950s, it was the number one killer, with little known as to how it happened.[2] Whilst we have been dealing with COVID-19 in the 21st century, heart disease was considered the epidemic of the 20th century.

During this time, in the small Pennsylvanian town of Roseto, lived a community of 1630 Italian immigrants and descendants. They had a relatively poor diet, rarely exercised and loved to smoke. Many of them had high blood pressure, diabetes and were obese. In other words, the people of Roseto had the same unhealthy habits and levels of risk factors associated with heart disease as everyone else in America.[3] The big difference was that they were not dying like everyone else. The average death rate in America from myocardial infarction was 3.5 males per thousand and 2.09 females. In Roseto it was 1 per thousand males and 0.6 thousand females.[4] That's a staggering 350% difference. How? Why? The story – and answer – is equal parts fascinating, bewildering and inspiring.

Emigration from Italy and immigration to America became somewhat free and easy towards the end of the 19th century when chunks of Italy were racked with poverty and tales of a better life existed in the United States. What started off with a small group of 11 emigrants ballooned to more than 1200 Italians leaving the small village of Roseto Valfortore in southern Italy and moving to America, eventually establishing and naming their own village in Roseto, Pennsylvania.[5]

It took time, but over many years the Rosetans implemented their Italian culture into their daily life in America. Much of the progress was led by the town's new priest, Pasquale de Nisco, who arrived in 1896 from London on a mission to elevate the standard of living in Roseto. His influence touched every part of daily life. He encouraged the townspeople to get American citizenship and bought land surrounding the church with a vision to build a plaza, cemetery, school and hospital.[6] He gave away seeds and bulbs and setup a community garden. He set up societies to encourage local sport, spiritual conversation and support of individuals and families during tough times. He set up a union and became president on behalf of the town's quarry workers, successfully doubling their wage. He encouraged the townspeople to setup businesses including bakeries and garment factories. He created a culture of cleanliness, organising rubbish removal and beautifying the town. He secured a liquor licence so the townspeople didn't need to leave their village to go to the bar with friends. Crime evaporated, the culture thrived, and the community of Roseto, Pennsylvania tread a path that would become the envy of America.[7]

On a summer's day in the late 1950s, American doctor Stewart Wolf gave a presentation to a local medical society in Pennsylvania. Wolf, who specialised in digestion and also taught at the University of Oklahoma, was invited to have a drink after the event by local doctor Benjamin Falcone. Falcone saw patients from Roseto and the neighbouring towns of Bangor and Nazareth. He shared with Wolf that over the duration of his 17 years as a local doctor, the incidence of heart attacks among Rosetans was extremely rare. Remember, this was at a time when heart disease was the nation's number one killer and cholesterol-lowering medications were decades away (statins weren't available until 1987).[8]

This was meat on a bone for Wolf, who gathered a team from the University to begin investigating. They checked birth and death certificates, doctors' records, took medical histories and lined up family trees. What started off as a preliminary four-week study located in the town council room became a summer-long investigation of the entire population of Roseto.

Wolf and his team got more than they bargained for. Mortality records showed that virtually no Rosetan under 55 had died of a heart attack and the death rate from heart disease was approximately 50% lower than the rest of the country.[9] For every 1000 men over 65, 10 Rosetans died from heart disease. In white America, it was over 19. In the neighbouring towns of Bangor and Nazareth it was more than 22 and 27 respectively.[10]

These results generated even more questions than answers, so Wolf dug deeper. He brought in colleague and sociologist, John Bruhn, to oversee interviews and they began hitting the pavement. The research team went from house to house and interviewed everyone over 21.

"They came to my house and asked me a lot of questions about my habits (such as), 'What do you eat?'" recalled one resident. "I think there were about 100 questions in the whole survey," said another. "I think everybody must have answered the same thing," according to a Rosetan woman featured in the TV docuseries *The Italian Americans*. "We ate everything wrong. We liked it! They (researchers) told us it was wrong. We didn't know it was wrong!"[11]

This is where it gets really interesting. It was clear diet and exercise was not to explain for the low death rate. But what was it? To find out if genetics was the key to their immunity, the researchers tracked down

350 relatives of the Rosetans who lived in the neighbouring villages and other parts of the US to determine if they had escaped the heart disease epidemic. They had not, dying in similar proportions to born and bred Americans.[12]

At this point it would have been easy to give up, throw the arms in the air, and walk away. But Wolf and Bruhn were determined to get their answers. And whilst walking down the streets of Roseto one day they realised that their answer was right in front of them.

The secret to Roseto was the Roseto way of life.

The researchers found families living with three and sometimes four generations under one roof. They found families dining together and giving leftovers to neighbours. They found old people dying of old age at home, surrounded by loved ones. In the town of Roseto no one was a stranger. During tough times the townspeople would rally to help the bereaved, sick and financially destitute. It was little wonder they could find hardly a trace of depression, drugs, suicide, alcoholism or crime.[13]

Think about that for a moment. How many communities do you know of where mental health, suicide, alcoholism, drugs and crime are not an issue? How many people do you know who have died of 'old age' or natural causes? It is now deemed so rare that 'natural causes' is no longer an official cause of death.

"The researchers did this extensive study and they came up with the bottom line," says Italian American author Adriana Trigiani.[14] "These people are not dying of heart attack because they feel emotionally safe. They're not afraid about old age because they're going to live with their families. They know they'll never starve because the guy next door has a garden and a cow. In this Italian American community, look how they live. They know *how* to live."[15]

The social structure in Roseto was the key difference and factor in its greater longevity and avoidance of heart disease. Not the Rosetan diet, not movement, nor a specific set of genes. Simply, the decision by Rosetans to connect with and care for each other was the secret to their robust heart health and longevity.

How to apply Roseto today

The story of Roseto exposes two elephants in the room. Firstly, it demonstrates that the health benefits of engaging with humanity, connecting with your community and celebrating your culture are completely understated and misunderstood. Secondly, Roseto is yet another reminder to avoid over-analysing diet. In a perhaps sad vindication of Wolf and Bruhn's research, the Roseto of today has lost its traditional lifestyle and its heart disease statistics are now in line with the rest of America.

So, before you jump on the next fad diet in the hope of a more exceptional life, consider the lessons of Roseto. Do you love your neighbours? Are you invested in your community? Are you cheerful to be around and generous by nature? For whilst Americans were counting their calories, watching their weight, and dying from heart disease, Rosetans were eating pizza, having dessert, and doing it with people they loved.

> *"Spaghetti is not the best thing for you all the time.*
> *But I tell you, if I'm going to go I'm going*
> *to go with a meatball in my mouth!"*
> **– Roseto resident during the Roseto study**

Connection is king

Roseto isn't an isolated study. Research from all over the planet and dating back to the 1940s shows that time and again, an active social life has powerful consequences. Smokers with active social lives live longer than anti-social non-smokers.[16] Pet owners with health conditions heal faster than those who live alone.[17] Socially engaged people suffer less depression and dementia. The consequences of loneliness are real and tangible. In addition, with the continued prevalence of mental illness and its link to social isolation, we know that loneliness – the absence of an empowering peer group – can even be fatal.

> **How would you rate the 'public spirit' of your community?**
> The English word 'community' derives from the Old French *comuneté*, which comes from the Latin *communitas* meaning 'community' or 'public spirit'. How would you rate the public spirit of the community you live in?

You Become Who You Hang Around

It's been said throughout the years that you are the average of the five people you spend the most time with. You'll have the average income of those five people, the average health, happiness, and almost anything else you measure. On face value most of us don't consider our peer group to be *that* influential. However when you write them down and really look at the results, it's difficult to argue with.

Who are the five people you spend the most time with? Write them down now on a piece of paper or put them in your phone. If you're a stay-at-home parent include your children. If you work long hours alongside others, then your colleagues are going to be in your top five. Depending on your lifestyle this list may include a mixture of your partner, children, work colleagues, friends, parents, and so on. It will depend on your stage of life, living arrangements, work situation and more.

For each person ask yourself:
1. Does this person support me in my dreams (no matter how wild your dreams may be)?
2. Does this person bring out the best in me?
3. Is it easy for me to be myself in front of this person?

Give a tick to each person who answers yes to all three questions. If that person does not get three ticks, mark a cross next to their name.

Admittedly, this top five list is a relatively simple exercise, but it's incredibly brutal. You may be itching to say "yeah but" and explain reasons why certain people who are unsupportive are on the list. If you prefer you can make two lists – one for your personal peer group and one for your professional peer group.

Whatever you decide, the list doesn't lie.

How to improve your peer group

Improving your peer group is one of the most challenging tasks in all areas of personal growth. It's also one of the most rewarding. Ask any person who left a violent relationship and you'll learn how difficult and equally freeing it can be. Depending on *who* it is that needs to come off your list will depend on how much time you spend procrastinating, avoiding or justifying their position on the list.

Family

Do you feel like you are being used as a crutch or platform for a family member to whinge, expand their victim story or even compare themselves to you? If so, it's time to heavily reduce your exposure to them and spend more time with empowering people.

It's fruitless to expect your family will *ever* change or adopt your point of view or way of life. Your family's role is not to agree with everything you do and understand all your decisions. More than anything, family is there to challenge you and help you grow. In many ways, when family members disagree with your point of view or way of life, the character-building and self-trust that is required is a great test of the decisions you are making.

Your job is to love your family, but that doesn't mean you are obliged to spend considerable amounts of time with them. Your family is the best personal growth course on the market. Almost every lesson you need to learn to live your exceptional life can be taught by your family. And entry is free! Seriously, if you can master your family relationships (which I define as unconditionally loving each person for who they are and not what they do or what they believe), you can more easily master the other key areas of life.

> *"Love your family; choose your peer group."*
> *– Tony Robbins*

Friends

Many people I work with have at least one friend where the relationship is more give than take. The friend is either needy, negative or simply disempowered in a way that doesn't make you inspired to spend time with them. You are loyal though and that's where the difficulty lies. Depending on the friendship, there are a number of ways to remove a friend from the top five.

1. *They don't call you and they don't return your calls.* If you are the one that constantly makes the calls to catch up, stop making the calls and see what happens. If you are not missed, it's a sign that the friendship was a one-way street. As brutal as it sounds, even our friends can fall into the socially acceptable trap of feeling 'too busy' to catch up, and so they'll never call us.
2. If you see a chronically disempowered friend regularly on a certain day and time of the week, decide to *do something that you love even more* at that time. Perhaps you want to do yoga, learn how to dance, speak a second language or learn an instrument, but you don't enrol because it conflicts with your social times. Bite the bullet and enrol. You're more likely to meet wonderful people when you do more of what you love and less of what you don't love. And as the saying goes, it's wiser to seek forgiveness rather than permission from your friend.
3. *Stop taking the calls.* This applies particularly to needy friends. If you've used your words and explained the inappropriateness of the constant contact, then there is often only one solution, and that is to let your actions do the talking. Generally speaking, needy friends were never taught by their parents how to be independent,

and essentially replace their parental relationships with their friends. If you're in one of those friendships, and it's becoming unbearable, then ripping off the band-aid is often the only solution.

Colleagues

Unsupportive colleagues can also be a difficult one, particularly if you love your work and have no intention of moving. Depending on the nature or hierarchy of the working relationship, understanding *why* your colleague's toxic behaviour exists is essential. Is their marriage falling apart, do they feel threatened by you, or is there some circumstance you're not aware of that's influencing their behaviour?

This book is not the forum to outline colleague relationship strategies in detail. Instead, I constantly recommend Dale Carnegie's *How To Win Friends and Influence People*.

The other relevant workplace scenario is if you feel unappreciated or undervalued. If you believe this will never change at your current employer, then there is really only one option to improve your life, and that is to leave. If you use an intimate relationship as an example, having an expectation that our partner will change is often fanciful and more than anything, completely out of our control. If you've appealed to the values of your workplace, done everything you can to communicate in their language and still find yourself unappreciated, start preparing the resignation letter.

Four ways to become a better friend

So far I've spoken about improving your own peer group. What happens though if you are a cross on someone else's list, or simply want to become a better friend? The art of friendship is rarely discussed and like many other parts of an exceptional social life, it quickly atrophies when we don't nurture it.

1. Spend at least 200 quality hours together

It's not outlandish to suggest good friendships take time to develop into exceptional ones. It might shock you though to find out how much *quality* time a great friendship requires. Jeffrey Hall, the Associate Professor of Communication Studies at the University of Kansas, found that it takes 50 hours of time together for an acquaintance to become a casual friend.[18] That's not working for your colleague for one week. Quality time is having lunch together, attending social functions and anything that is more personal than professional. It takes 90 hours to go from casual friend to general friend status, and more than 200 hours before you consider someone your close friend.[19]

"We have to put that time in," Hall said. "You can't snap your fingers and make a friend. Maintaining close relationships is the most important work we do in our lives – most people on their deathbeds agree."

If you have a look at the top five people you hang around, how much quality time have you spent with them? If it's very little, it's unlikely you feel safe to confide your biggest fears or your greatest dreams to them or anyone. The remedy is as simple as it is difficult. Prioritising quality time with others in the short-term is the only way to create a sense of belonging, community, confidence and connection in the long-term.

2. Talk about your problems

In the 1980s, 86 women with terminal metastatic breast cancer were split into two groups by Dr David Spiegel and his research team at Stanford Medical School.[20] All 86 women were receiving the same medical treatment, but one group attended weekly support meetings.

Imagine 43 women sitting in a circle expressing their emotions for 90 minutes each week. They were encouraged to express their fears, anger, anxiety and so on. What impact do you think this would have on their physical health?

The impact was extraordinary. The women in the support group had *twice* the survival time of women in the control group. The women in the support group lived an average of 37 months after entering the program, compared to 19 months for the control group.

The support group also experienced less mood swings, physical pain and fear than the control group. Incredibly, when Spiegel delivered his findings 12 years later, three of the 86 (remember they were all considered terminal) were still alive, and they were the ones who were the *most socially active* within the group.[21]

Please note, you do *not* need to have breast cancer to share your problems, fears and anxieties. When you release your emotions, you not only create a bond with people, you massively improve your physical health at the same time.

This is particularly important for people eating the 'perfect' diet. I've worked with thousands of people who eat so well, yet have toxic relationships in the home or workplace and are too fearful to do anything about it. They have no emotional connection with their partner or their colleagues, and despite a great diet (and maybe even exercise), they still have serious physical symptoms. This may present as an autoimmune disease or digestive complaint, and on an emotional level can present as major anxiety or depression.

3. Be there in the tough times

When I was 18 one of my best friends developed testicular cancer. Jacob was a family friend and 23 at the time. I regularly visited Jacob at the hospital, particularly during the tough times of chemotherapy when he was in major pain. He looked so different. Completely bald, white as a ghost and often writhing in so much pain, I couldn't help to just squeeze his hand and tell him to hang in there.

About two years later, a cancer-free Jacob was recounting those days and shared with me just how much he valued my friendship and presence during those dark days. I didn't quite know what he meant or why he said it until he told me that his school friends had effectively deserted him during this time. He wasn't bitter about it, as he knew just how difficult it would have been for young men in their 20s to be reminded of their mortality. Over the years this experience has stuck with me as a reminder to be there for friends in the fun *and* the frightening times.

"Everyone wants to ride with you in the limo," says Oprah Winfrey. "But what you want is someone who will take the bus with you when the limo breaks down." In longevity cultures, lifelong friends are there through thick *and* thin. They are there to celebrate birth *and* grieve death. They are there to help you celebrate your children's weddings *and* your parent's funerals. It's easy to be there to celebrate the good times. The question is, as a friend, do you go missing when your friends need you more than ever?

4. Help without seeking permission

When my auntie Maureen died in 2016 I gave my grieving cousin Carly a hug and said: "If there's anything I can do just let me know." Carly and I are close so when she said to me, "I hate it when people say that," I was both taken aback and all ears.

Carly's view, and I completely agree, is that a grieving or struggling person doesn't need that kind of open-ended support. Grieving people don't need to be asking you to make a meal or pick up the kids from school. Instead, grieving people just love it when you *do* something for them without asking.

I think most of us love this too, whether we are grieving or not. We love things being done for us because someone *thought* of us. In other words, someone showed love for us. Telling someone you'll do anything for them, without being specific, is essentially a throwaway line to be polite. Our friends deserve more than that from us.

> ### Exceptional Exercise 3.1: Be the exceptional friend
> Who is struggling, grieving or unwell in your world right now? Just go and do something for them without asking. Make them a meal, pick their kids up from school, take their children for a day, run errands for them, mow their lawns or book a cleaner for their house. Anything! No permission needed. Just do it.

The magic of the moai

Women from the island of Okinawa in Japan live an average of eight years longer than American women.[22] One reason is undoubtedly their exceptional social life, which has its foundation with their peer group known as a *moai* (mo-eye).

Moai roughly translates in English to 'meeting for a common purpose'. When Okinawan children are young, they are paired together with four others to form the moai. They were originally formed as a way of financially supporting a village. If someone needed money to buy land or an emergency situation arose (illness, environmental, etc), the only way to finance it was often to aggregate money locally. Over the years, the moai ethos has broadened to become a social support network and foundation for companionship.

Members of the moai meet for life, with some meeting daily to gossip, talk about life, offload stress, give or receive advice and, when required, provide financial assistance.

In all longevity cultures, social connectedness is an embedded part of the lifestyle. Is it an embedded part of yours? You don't need to relocate your life in order to cultivate this exceptional social life, but if you do want to add years to your life, you simply must make some friends. Sporting and recreational clubs, cafes and places of worship are just some examples of where you might find or create a moai.

Why and how I uprooted my life

My wife was in tears. Life had become one stressful ticking time bomb waiting to explode. It was late 2012, and Sarah had spent more than two years attempting to balance motherhood and work, and it was creating emotional turmoil. Life wasn't meant to be so unfun. One night, Sarah was standing in the living room crying from sheer exhaustion. "I just can't do it anymore. I'm so tired," she told me. I was standing in front of her, taking in the sorrow and sadness she felt, when I found myself saying: "Let's just sell up and move! You don't deserve to be so sad babe. This is not what life is all about. We don't have to struggle through life this way."

Sarah's eyes widened in a mixture of shock and possibility.

"We can't possibly sell," was her first response. Hundreds of people relied on Sarah for her incredible chiropractic care and that overwhelming sense of responsibility was a burden Sarah struggled to let go of. But the idea of releasing it was also mentally, emotionally and spiritually intoxicating for Sarah. The opportunity to be a stay-at-home mum was not just a dream for Sarah, it was a calling she was having a hard time suppressing.

In our six years in Inverloch, we had never felt the urge to buy a family home. And whilst we had casual friends, we definitely didn't have close friends. In our travels in 2006 we had spent a day together in Byron Bay and had one of those beautifully romantic days when everything flowed. The sun was shining, the food was incredible, the beach was idyllic and the people were so friendly. It felt somewhat utopian at the time and it stayed that way for years, until we decided we wanted to leave Inverloch.

We had always wanted to live by the coast instead of inland. Inverloch had provided that, except six winters there showed us that we definitely craved a warmer climate. With two young children and school on the horizon, we also decided that a Rudolf Steiner school would be a key part of our lifestyle and community for the next two decades. We mapped out the locations of Steiner schools on the east coast of Australia, and zeroed in on Byron Bay to Noosa. Before making a final decision on where our family's future lay, we went on a week-long reconnaissance trip to Byron.

We arrived in September 2013, fortuitously in the same week as the Spring Fair for one of the local Steiner schools. Getting a glimpse into school life gave us great confidence that we had not only found the little piece of Australia we wanted to live in, we had found our community and the foundation for the next chapter of our own exceptional lives.

We never made it to Noosa. Instead, we stayed in Byron Bay for the week, immersing ourselves as much as possible to ensure we were making the best decision, and then went home to sell our business.

When you make a big decision that feels right, there'll be moments of incredible synchronicity and moments of seemingly insurmountable challenge. The challenges exist to test out how badly you really want it.

Our business sold effortlessly which was a huge relief. With a timeline now firm, Sarah and I went up to Byron for two nights to look at six or seven rental properties. We were determined to live in Byron Bay for all the buzz and easy access to the lifestyle we thought we wanted. It didn't turn out that way though. Every property we viewed was not suitable for a variety of reasons, and at the end of day one, Sarah was in tears.

The following day, we headed to the Mullumbimby farmers market and got chatting to a number of locals who suggested other towns surrounding Byron Bay. These were areas we'd never looked at (or even heard of) such was our tunnel-vision tourist mindset. Thanks to a community whose culture oozed generosity and care, we now had more options and within a matter of two hours we had inspected a property and signed a lease. We boarded the flight back to Victoria knowing where we'd be based for the beginning of our next chapter. Smooth sailing? No way. A rollercoaster? Definitely. Worth it? Absolutely.

Resist the resistance

You might be reading this and recognise you don't truly connect with your community. You don't have many (or any) close friends nearby, you're not drawn to any meeting places, sporting or special interest groups, and you lack any local patriotism or pride for the area you live in.

If this is you, you have two options –
1. Take a good hard look at yourself. If you are going to uproot your entire life, you have to truly ask yourself if the problem is you or your community. If you're not connecting with people, is it because you're not making the effort? Will you be taking the same social baggage with you to a new community? Before you commit to leaving, it's wise to give your community every opportunity to connect.
2. Leave town for a community you love to live in. If you've engaged fully in your community and you know it's time to leave, you're in for a wild ride. Starting over is not easy and it's not something I recommend unless you have a genuine pull to move. But if you're

prepared for the lows of the rollercoaster as well as the highs, moving to a community where you love to live just may be the wisest decision you ever make in life.

> *"Somehow we've come to equate success with not needing anyone. Many of us are willing to extend a helping hand, but we're very reluctant to reach out for help when we need it ourselves. It's as if we've divided the world into 'those who offer help' and 'those who need help'. The truth is that we are both."*
> *– Brené Brown*

🔺 🔺 🔺

Time, Social Media and Green Grass

None of us are without time. In fact, time is the only thing we have. Time is the great leveler of life, each of us having been given 24 hours per day to spend. And the brutal truth is that we spend this time according to our highest priorities. When you or someone else says you don't have time to do something or see someone, the translation is "there is something I value more importantly than this." We just prefer to say it more politely. If you're in back-to-back meetings all day, you might tell your friend "I don't have time" to have lunch, but really you're saying that the meetings are more important than the lunch. If an emergency occurred, you'd cancel the meetings and tend to the emergency, because that was more important. It's never a question of time, it's always a question of priorities. *I don't have time* is nothing more than a socially-acceptable excuse and all excuses are veiled lies disguised to keep the other person from being offended.

What makes an exceptional social life even more elusive for many is the culturally accepted lifestyle that prioritises work, Netflix and social media over authentic socialising. So precious and novel has authentic human-to-human contact become that we now have the hashtag #IRL (in real life) for it.

Behind the lie of *I don't have time* is the truth that an exceptional social life is one of the greatest ways to *increase* your productivity. For example, if you find yourself regularly working late in the office, setting up a social 'appointment' for 6 or 7pm is the best thing you can do for yourself. It will force you to put your tools down and recharge for the next day. From inviting friends over for dinner to visiting your parents each week, attending yoga with a friend or reconnecting with schoolmates, adding the vibrancy of an exceptional social life provides you with an added layer of richness that nothing else can.

Socialising for extroverts and introverts is different

What is becoming increasingly clear is that extroverts and introverts socialise very differently. In her book *Quiet Impact*, Sylvia Loehken imagines extroverts as wind turbines and introverts as batteries.[23] Whilst both require human interaction for survival, their energy is created very differently. Extroverts *generate* energy from their social interactions – they require social situations to actually start the wind turbine spinning and they also require human contact to keep their energy up. Introverts on the other hand wake up with a full battery that is unplugged as soon as they hop out of bed. Social interactions will lower the battery's reserves – some situations more than others – and the introvert will then need quiet time to recharge. In an excruciating cosmic joke for many, introverts and extroverts often fall in love with each other and equally are attracted to friends who display their socially opposite behaviour.

If you're an introvert it's likely you're looking for a few deep, genuine friendships that could last a lifetime. If you're an extrovert (which I am), having a large number of casual friends and acquaintances is likely to come naturally to you.

As a result, socialising is energising for the extroverts and for the introverts it can be enriching; when done with the *right* people. On the flipside, beware the energy vampires who suck all the life out of you with 'stinking thinking' and sob stories. You know who I'm talking about and you know how you feel when you spend too much time with them. As I said at the beginning of this chapter, you become who you hang around, so be very careful who you spend your precious time with.

Social media is not socialising

Whilst over 40% of the global population is on social media platforms including Facebook, Instagram, Twitter, Tik Tok and WeChat, it's easy for people to confuse social media with socialising. On average we spend two hours and 22 minutes each day on social media, giving rise to a belief that we are becoming a more social world.[24] I find next to nothing, however, to suggest that we are becoming better at socialising. At the core of socialising is body language and two-way verbal communication; reading cues and engaging in the art of conversation is sadly dying amongst all generations who prioritise social media over socialising.

Dale Carnegie's iconic *How To Win Friends And Influence People* now has an updated version for the digital age, such is the impact of technology on our social skills. Being able to socialise effectively is like a muscle. The more we do it the stronger we get, and the more different settings we place ourselves in, the more adaptable we become. If the majority of our human connection is spent in front of a computer or a screen, our social muscle atrophies and withers. The result is an inclination to avoid social settings, making it difficult to connect with our community. Gone is the belief that 'a stranger is a friend we haven't met yet,' replaced with 'stranger danger'. How can we improve our social lives living on such high alert?

If we were to give back just half our social media consumption and increase our human connection, share our feelings more, listen to others with compassion and master the art of being ourselves around others, we would not only bring more grace to humanity, we would find our daily lives much more fulfilling and simply easier.

At the same time, social media is not to blame for people becoming socially disengaged. "Social media is neutral," Dr John Demartini behavioural expert shared with me on *100 Not Out*. "It's ...or evil, positive or negative. It's merely a technology to ...uman behaviour. You can use it to create your virtues or vice. ... can use it to share your love and advice. It depends on how it's used."

How are you using social media? Is it feeding your deepest desires or your darkest fears? Giving up on social media is not the answer; instead ensure it's enhancing your life, enriching your friendships and being controlled *by* you rather than controlling you.

"Are we recording?" The grace of consistency

One of the more profound observations I had as a radio and television producer was the emotional volatility of some presenters. Their off-air persona would completely change when the red recording light came on as if they were acting in a movie. Many colleagues had a personality that remained consistent whether they were recording or not, however I observed that the presenters my colleagues complained about regularly were the ones who were most volatile. These presenters were hard to work with, kicking and screaming or being aloof one minute and then behaving like an angel the next.

We can all be two-faced sometimes. Many of us lead split lives, with different personality traits required in the workplace compared to the family home. The challenge that the *Exceptionals* have mastered is having consistency, most of the time. Being similar 'on the air' as 'off the air' is one of the most powerful social traits you can master. When your personality in the home is similar to your personality *out* of the home, you'll have more energy to be present with people rather than toiling to be 'on show' every time you walk out the front door. That will exhaust you and is largely inauthentic. You can fake a smile all day long, but you also resist help and support when you're pretending everything is fine when it's anything but.

The grass is never greener

Crisis teaches people that 'stuff' doesn't matter; human beings do. Death is a great reminder that all the cars, fancy houses and labels will not bring you fulfilment in the long-term. "I don't care what my neighbour has," Eddie Jaku shared with me on *100 Not Out*. "I don't know the troubles he has. Maybe he has more money, but it doesn't matter. My car is a tool to take me from A to B. I don't care if my neighbour drives a Rolls Royce. This is not important in life. What's important is your surroundings and your family. Yes, you must strive to have a nice house, but it doesn't have to be a castle. We are not born with castles. Our ancestors lived in little caves."

Rather than attempting to keep up with your peer group, heed the advice of Jaku and *The Exceptionals* by developing relationships without ambition or agenda. "I enjoy catching up with my friends to have a coffee and some cake, too! This satisfaction is like medicine," Jaku says. "This is why, thank God, I look good, I feel good (and) I walk fast. When people ask me: 'Why do you walk so fast?' I say: 'When you're my age you don't know how long you have!' This is what life is all about. It's not the big things. The big things you cannot change. It's the little things that make you happy."

What is your social medicine? Is it material possessions, news or social media – short-term gratifying drugs that have a never-ending appetite? Or is it your peer group? Time and again, *The Exceptionals* show us that spending time with people who care about you will remedy most, if not all, your ills. You don't need to keep up with the Kardashians, the Joneses, or anyone else you're easily jealous of. You need to simply follow the script of *Your Exceptional Life* and avoid reading the juicy (and often factually incorrect) bits of everyone else's.

> *"A man's growth is seen in the successive choirs of his friends."*
> **– Ralph Waldo Emerson**

PART TWO

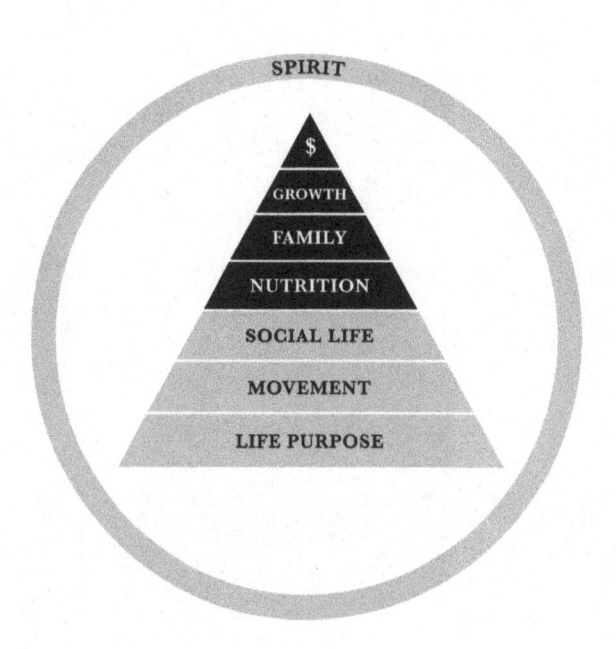

YOUR
EXCEPTIONAL
QUALITY OF LIFE

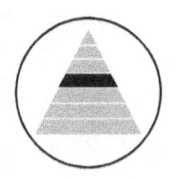

NUTRITION

"To eat is a necessity, but to eat intelligently is an art."
– Francois de la Rochefoucauld

Is it a cosmic joke that many diet gurus die prematurely? Or is it a sign that perhaps food is not the fountain of youth, vitality and longevity many mistake it to be? Surely, if diet were the most important factor in living a great, long life, the healthy eaters would live the longest?

On the flipside, the sad reality is that obesity is causing 44% of diabetes and 40% of many cancers.[1] Exceptional nutrition therefore requires a new philosophy, and it lives in the shared experiences of *The Exceptionals*, both past and present. This chapter is dedicated to unpacking Rochefoucauld's mantra. *The Exceptionals* are not fine-dining snobs. They are not at the cutting edge of nutrition, well-read on the latest superfood or antioxidant.

There is no one *Exceptional* diet, and our ancestors left more dietary clues than modern day food gurus. Eating intelligently is not exclusively focused on *what* to eat. Instead, mastering the art of nutrition requires a shift in thinking to also include *how* to eat, *why* we eat and *who* to eat with. In addition, beverage consumption is an art, and too many of us have demoted our tea, coffee and alcohol to mere stimulants or tranquillising drugs. Reclaiming the magic and true purpose of what we eat and drink will unshackle the rigid foodie and yo-yo dieter alike.

If mediocrity persists with nutrition, the consequences become unbearable and often fatal. The overly exceptional eater who develops social anxiety suffers the same consequences as the obese diabetic. Friendships and family relationships are strained, bank balances are exhausted, careers become stifled and souls are crushed. Being too exceptional is not better than the everyday average diet. A happy medium, which *The Exceptionals* are all too good at finding, is the only way forward for an exceptional life to be realised.

When you connect your nutrition to your life purpose and see how mastering the art of eating intelligently benefits all areas of your exceptional life, you'll quit counting calories and worrying about your genes. Instead you'll find a sustenance, energy and level of inspiration you never knew existed. But first we must address how we got into this hot mess of disease and disaster in the first place.

▲ ▲ ▲

Sick, Fat and Malnourished

I mentioned it in the introduction to this section and it bears repeating again. According to the World Health Organization, obesity is responsible for 44% of all diabetes and 40% of 13 forms of cancer.[2] When you consider the aforementioned statistic from Professor Michael Woodward that physical inactivity causes 42% of all dementia on the planet, one can't help but feel aghast and embarrassed at the simplicity of the solution and equal magnitude of the problem.

For years society has connected overweight and obesity with high blood pressure, high cholesterol and diabetes, but cancer and dementia have rarely been linked to what you eat and how you move. Sadly, obesity is seen as something that we can tolerate without ever having to do too much about. We can still work, rest and play and live life like many others, until the impending diagnosis and eventual lowered quality of life appears.

Obesity can cause cancer of the esophagus, pancreas, colon, breast (after menopause), endometrium, kidney, thyroid and gallbladder among others.[3] Living an exceptional life whilst obese is possible, but as mentioned the consequences of mediocrity in just one area of life can be and often are disastrous for all other areas of life.

Cancer is the perfect case in point. Work, wealth and family are three obvious pillars that can fall apart during a cancer diagnosis. At the same time, crises of this kind can be the making of many. More than anything, these very real statistics put the responsibility on the individual to improve, and most people are not prepared to take a position of leadership for their health. It is much easier to take insulin for diabetes and conventional drugs for cancer than to proactively deal with the obesity. I'm not suggesting to avoid insulin or conventional medicine in certain situations; what is clear though is that obesity doesn't occur from a lack of insulin, and cancer isn't the result of an absence of drugs.

The doctor won't make you well, the dietician won't make you slim and the personal trainer won't make you fit. The work can only be done by you. Looking for a saviour your entire life will not only send you crazy; the chase for the silver bullet will completely disempower you.

"People looking for the magic bullet usually get shot."
– Dr John Demartini

The hard facts on fat
- Worldwide obesity has nearly tripled since 1975.
- In 2016, more than 1.9 billion adults, 18 and older, were overweight.
- Of these, 650 million were obese.
- 39% of adults aged 18 and over were overweight in 2016, and 13% were obese.
- 65% of the world's population live in countries where overweight and obesity kills more people than underweight.
- 41 million children under the age of 5 were overweight or obese in 2016.
- More than 340 million children and adolescents aged 5–19 were overweight or obese in 2016.
- Obesity is preventable.

Source: World Health Organization[4]

We are dying from diseases of nutritional extravagance

More than 14 million people die each year from *diseases of poverty* (including AIDS/HIV, malaria, tuberculosis, diarrhea and measles).[5] Diseases of poverty are often communicable (infectious) diseases, with malnutrition often a ubiquitous or co-morbid factor. Diseases of affluence claim the lives of more than 40 million people each year and are *not* infectious.[6] Instead, diseases of affluence are often caused by personal lifestyles and an increase of wealth in society. In other words, if you've never worried about where your next meal will come from or if you'll have a roof over your head, you live in a country of affluence where sanitation, food and shelter are not the threat to your mortality. Instead, it's more likely that your lifestyle is the predator.

Diseases of affluence have also been referred to as diseases of 'nutritional extravagance' by Cornell University Professor and author of *The China Study*, Dr Thomas Colin Campbell. Our affluence has created malnutrition of a different kind – excessive junk food, large portions, second and third helpings are all problems that are within our control. And yet meal by meal, day by day, year by year, we add a toxic load to our body that in time manifests as a disease of affluence.

> **Top 10 causes of death in affluent countries**
> According to the World Health Organization (WHO) the top 10 causes of death in affluent countries in 2016 were from:
> 1. Ischemic heart diseases
> 2. Stroke
> 3. Alzheimer's disease and other dementia
> 4. Trachea, bronchus and lung cancer
> 5. Chronic obstructive pulmonary disease
> 6. Lower respiratory infections
> 7. Colon and rectum cancers
> 8. Diabetes
> 9. Kidney diseases
> 10. Breast cancer
>
> Except for the lower respiratory infections all of the above are non-communicable diseases. In 2016 WHO reported 56.9 million deaths worldwide, and more than half (54%), were due to the above causes.

Source: World Health Organization[7]

Dosage is the killer

Whilst doctors take the Hippocratic Oath to 'first do no harm', most of us have forgotten to make that oath to ourselves. One of the key fundamentals of the healing arts is dosage, for as Swiss physician Paracelsus declared in the 16th century, it is: "The dose that makes the poison. All things are poison, and nothing is without poison, the dosage alone makes it so a thing is not a poison." No chemical is immune from this – too much water will drown just as too little will dehydrate. Both dosages cause death.

What is so obvious yet perhaps too close to our eyes to see is that our lifetime dosage of food – much of it poorly grown and produced, poorly eaten and poorly digested – is contributing greatly to our diseases of affluence – often first showing up as excess weight, high blood pressure or high cholesterol with a cascade of diseases following.

We need to learn to be our own doctor and nutritionist, in charge of the dosage and medicine – which is the food we put in our mouths each and every day of our lives. We can no longer afford to live by the mantra of 'everything in moderation'. Society has completely misinterpreted its meaning, choosing to focus more on the word *everything* than *moderation*. Moderation translates to being temperate, mild or controlled. We are anything but mild or controlled when it comes to our diet. Instead, our actions – and our death rates – show that we have become an 'everything to excess' society, and our extravagance is killing us in droves.

In contrast, longevity cultures and *The Exceptionals* – who also proclaim the 'everything in moderation' philosophy – focus more on the word *moderation* than *everything*. The Okinawans practise *hara hachi bu* – eating until they are 80% full – the Ikarians frown upon getting drunk, whilst everyday *Exceptionals* you and I have never met eat simply rather than extravagantly. If your ancestors grew up through wars, rations or hard times of any kind – they were forced to, and often continued to, eat temperately and eat to live rather than live to eat.

▲ ▲ ▲

What Then, Shall We Eat?

There is a disturbing trend in the diet industry. Robert Atkins, founder of the Atkins Diet, died at 72 from a heart attack. Nathan Pritikin, founder of the Pritikin Diet (dubbed "the healthiest diet on earth"), developed two forms of leukemia before committing suicide aged 69.

Michael Montignac, a diet developer who founded the Montignac Diet and influenced the South Beach Diet, died of prostate cancer aged 66.

Adelle Davis, known as 'the most famous nutritionist of the early to mid-20th century', died aged 70 from cancer. Davis claimed it was caused by the junk food she ate in her younger years and a series of x-rays she underwent.

If we are what we eat, surely the diet gurus would be sitting at the top of the longevity ladder? Clearly, life as a human being is more complicated than the food that passes our lips.

We're becoming just like diet experts

This premature death or tunnel-vision on diet is not exclusive to the diet experts. I've observed many people that make their diet too exceptional at the expense of the other key pillars of life.

Visualise this: Mary is eating a pasture-raised open-range chicken salad at her workstation or in the kitchen. It is organic, locally sourced and contains no artificial flavours or preservatives. She is very proud of herself because she is doing the 'right' thing. The diet experts would give Mary a big pat on the back and proclaim she is well on the way to a long and healthy life because 'we are what we eat'. Mary though, also hates her job, rarely moves her body (believing that eating well is more important than moving well), doesn't socialise with her friends because they 'don't understand' her or she has 'no time', and finds herself growing apart from her husband because he 'doesn't understand' her either. The only books she reads are on nutrition, and like most people she spends more than she earns. Her religion is food and she can't understand why people 'don't understand' that. She's right, they're wrong.

Sadly I'm not exaggerating here. Whilst not all elements of that example apply to everyone, our food choices have become an identity that consumes so much of our thoughts that we've lost perspective on what is truly important in life. Drinking green juices, being gluten-free or vegan and eating a strictly organic and biodynamic diet are all wonderful – yet none are the foundation of an exceptional life.

No one diet is the answer

When National Geographic sent Dan Buettner and his team around the planet in search of the world's longest-lived people, they didn't find that one diet fits all. The European Blue Zones of Ikaria and Sardinia eat a Mediterranean diet including vegetables, fruit, herbs, bread, olive oil and wine. Their regular intake of gluten, grains, sugar and alcohol flies in the face of the gluten-free, grain-free and strict vegan diet approaches.

In Loma Linda, California, there is a population of Seventh Day Adventists outliving their countrymen and women and most of the world. Most Loma Lindans are vegetarian, whilst some are strict vegan.[8] Further south, in the Blue Zone of Nicoya, Costa Rica, they subsist largely on corn, eggs, rice, beans, wild fruits and vegetables. In Okinawa their traditional diet includes plenty of rice, fish, tofu, vegetables, and very little fruit.

What these cultures have in common is just as intriguing as what they don't. Moreover, what their diets teach us is that there is no one way of eating that suits the globe's entire population. With that in mind then, the question still remains, what do you eat?

> *"People have to find their own way and then everybody has to leave everybody else alone with whatever they're doing because we're all trying to do our best to stay healthy. For me I do my best being all raw."*
> **– Mimi Kirk**

The seven-word diet

What any culture, across any time can agree on and adjust to from season to season is Michael Pollan's seven word answer to the question of what the best diet is for human beings. Outlined in more detail in his little masterpiece *Food Rules*, Pollan uses these seven words to summarise his findings –

Eat food. Mostly plants. Not too much.

Let that sink in for a minute. Ikarians and Sardinians don't pile the respective goat and lamb on to the plate first and leave a small space for some tomatoes and cucumber. Okinawans don't pile the fish or rice on top of a small serving of vegetables. Instead, they acknowledge that plants are the foundation of their diet – the basis for their food intake – but not the exclusive and only component of their diet. They eat real food, not junk disguised as food; and they know when to stop eating, so they're not dying from diseases of nutritional extravagance.

When in doubt look to your ancestors

Some years ago, my *100 Not Out* co-host, Damian Kristof, was assessing a patient who had decided to go on a low-carbohydrate, grain-free, sugar-free, dairy-free paleolithic diet. She was perplexed that she had put on weight, had developed red and cracking skin, and didn't experience the energy the paleo diet leaders said she would. When Damian quizzed her on what she'd been eating, her answer included a lot of coconut products including coconut oil, desiccated coconut, coconut water, coconut cream and coconut milk.

When Damian asked where her ancestry lay, the woman explained that it was predominantly Irish. "How many coconut trees do you see in Ireland?" Damian quizzed with a cheeky grin on his face. Instantly the woman knew what he meant. She had not been observing the importance of her ancestry as a clue to define her ideal diet, and she is not alone. Instead of checking our family tree or reading the book of our family history, we're reading the book of a nutritionist, or scarier still, an unqualified guru who has no idea about you, your body, your history, or your lifestyle.

I have ancestral ties back to Scotland, England, Germany and Lebanon, so a diet rich in Indian food is perhaps not going to serve me best. If you have no ancestral or genetic connection to Asia, then it's likely that a high consumption of soy will not be beneficial. This is not to say that Indian or Asian food is *bad* for you and I, but just like the Irish woman who made coconut products a large part of her diet, we must be careful not to make genetically foreign foods a foundational part of our food intake.

What all diets have in common

Whether you're observing the longevity cultures or the latest diet craze, what all diets have in common is simple and wise. No sensible diet recommends moderate amounts of lollies, soft drinks, fast food products, bags of chips, fried food, heavily processed alcohol and packaged foods.

In addition, all mainstream diets have a strong focus on fruits and vegetables. What differentiates most diets is the source and amount consumed of each macronutrient – protein, carbohydrates and fat. This is the sticking point and source of debate amongst the diet gurus and evangelical eaters. Do you choose animal protein or plant-based protein? Do you focus on complex carbs, starchy carbs or simple sugars? What type of fats do you consume?

Your job is to work out (largely through trial and error and observing your ancestry) what the ideal mix is for you. What I do know is *The Exceptionals* don't spend their time weighing their meals, observing menus with painstaking precision and measuring out their proportions of protein, carbohydrates and fat. Don't blindly follow the diet experts or your friends and expect the same results; instead listen to your body and observe the wisdom it provides you.

Eat SLOWER ... most of the time

Once you've considered your ancestry, the next step is to observe what grows around you and cultivate a diet largely based on your local environment. Longevity cultures and many *Exceptionals* have a philosophy, conscious or not, that is to eat –

- Seasonal
- Local
- Organic
- Wholefoods
- Ethical, Environmental, Economical
- Regenerative

And most importantly, they live by this philosophy *most* of the time and not all of the time. *The Exceptionals* will have a piece of cake at a birthday party, a beer with friends, or some ice cream with their grandchildren. But these 'sometimes' foods are simply that; food they eat only sometimes and are not the foundation of their food intake. *Exceptionals* understand that their body is robust enough to enjoy these foods *some of the time* without suffering any long-term consequences.

Seasonal: Go to any local farmers market and you can be rest assured the produce is seasonal (otherwise it wouldn't be there). Personally, I couldn't tell you when certain fruits and vegetables are in season, but what I can tell you is that I go to the farmers market each Tuesday and buy whatever I want, knowing that all the produce is fresh and in season. I see Rod for my kale and herbs, Denise for my lettuce, Heather for my tomatoes, cucumbers, capsicum and zucchini, Jesse for my potatoes and eggplant and Kate for my avocados. If Kate's not there, I know that avocados aren't in season. Some years Kate is there for eight weeks, whereas other years it could be six weeks or 12 weeks. Every season yields different amounts of avocados.

When you go to the supermarket, it's far harder to know what is in season and what isn't – because everything is available. If you live far away from a farmers market, I suggest you shop at your local green grocer and ask questions about what is in season and local. Price is often a good indicator – in-season foods are often at their lowest price as supply is so high.

Local: Food miles is a measure outlining how far your food has travelled from its original location. Shortly after moving from Melbourne to Byron Bay, I realised just how plentiful the macadamia nut was in our local region. We had, however, brought our regular shopping habits up from Victoria and continued to buy cashews regularly. One day whilst making a smoothie I observed that the organic cashews were from Ecuador. It seemed silly that we were buying cashews from a country 15,432 kilometres away when we had incredible nuts growing in our proverbial backyard. We made a decision then and there to only buy macadamias and Australian-grown nuts and to cease buying imported nuts.

When you eat seasonally and local, supporting your local economy will bring even more fulfilment to your meals. When you know the people who have contributed to your delicious dinner or Christmas lunch, you'll enrich the connection you have to your plate and also eat it more consciously.

"Most of us know who our doctor is," explains regenerative farmer, Charlie Arnott. "We see them once or twice a year for a checkup. But if I ask you 'who is your farmer?' most of us wouldn't have a clue. Most people don't know a farmer. Yet how often do you depend on a farmer? For many it's three times a day."

Arnott has a point. When you consider all the food you buy, how much of it is from people you know personally? Whilst traditional cultures have a strong relationship with their land and the people who grow food, most in society don't know a single person who personally grows the food they eat.

Organic: Organic doesn't need to be certified organic. Given the often-unreasonable costs of organic food, homegrown produce is often better than certified organic. If the food grew in the local environment it probably didn't need any interference to go from a seed to a crop. Not all of the stands I visit at the farmers market are certified organic, but I know they've grown their food to perhaps even higher standards than the organic certification requires. It's always wise to ask if crops have been sprayed, and if you're satisfied with the answer, you're better off purchasing a local, home-grown apple than a certified organic one from another country.

Wholefood: Keeping food as close to its original form is a key factor for longevity cultures around the world. Whilst some people might say that there's apple in an apple pie (so it must be healthy), traditional cultures are more likely to simply eat the apple or stew the apple. Processing is a natural and normal part of human life and is not to be avoided; it's the level of processing that has become the new normal in society that we must be wary of. Eating a wholefood diet means you can pronounce your ingredients, locate them easily, and prepare the meal from scratch without relying on any synthetic additives.

Ethical: Society is littered with many shades of grey when it comes to ethical standards. From farming practices to modern slavery and the processing of plant-based proteins to treatment of animals, there are a number of factors that make up the ethics of our food choices. Without attempting to regurgitate the different ethical views in this book, it's important to eat in a way that *you* feel is ethical – and to allow others to eat in a way that *they* believe is ethical.

Environmental: There are significant arguments to suggest conventional agricultural practices are having a disastrous effect on our environment, let alone the death of the animal. At the same time, there is an equally valid argument to suggest lab-made fake meat is equally unethical and unnatural for humanity. What can't be ignored is the disastrous and largely avoidable impact food waste is having on the planet.[9]

One third of all food produced globally is lost or wasted every year. This equates to 1.3 billion tonnes of waste in landfill (more than 2.3 million Olympic-size swimming pools). Beyond shameful is the environmental impact of uneaten food. If global food waste were a country, it would be the world's third biggest greenhouse gas emitter behind USA and China. Food waste causes 8% of greenhouse gases heating the planet. Just as, if not more alarming is the humanitarian cost of our global food waste. Almost 800 million people are undernourished, yet if just 25% of food waste could be saved, 870 million people would be fed.[10]

Economical: From the perspective of food waste, the average Australian wastes $3800 per year on uneaten food.[11] That's a very good holiday thrown in to the bin each year!

We are our own mini restaurant, and many *Exceptionals*, particularly those who have experienced war rations, recessions and hard times, know the importance of being economical with food. When you consider that day after day, three main meals turns into more than 1,000 meals per year, there is nothing stingy or tightfisted with being economical with your food (especially given the environmental impact our over-abundance and wastage is creating).

Regenerative: We have been living in a growing agrochemical world since the mid 1800s. Led by behemoths Bayer, Monsanto and Syngenta, herbicides, fungicides, insecticides, fertilisers and all types of weed killers (think Roundup) have been liberally sprayed upon the paddocks and gardens of farmers and green thumbs alike for well over a century.

From droughts and floods to bushfires and melting ice, humanity's awareness of conventional agriculture's deleterious effects is causing a major shift. Documentaries including David Attenborough's *A Life On Our Planet* and Damon Gameau's *2040* demonstrate just how impactful the planet's mass clearing of land is on the environment.

This global movement to replenish our planet is being led by consumers, farmers and food producers, and the core of that transition is from conventional to regenerative agriculture. This 'back to the future' method of farming and feeding humanity is an approach based on conservation and rehabilitation of the land. The benefits of regenerative farming include topsoil regeneration, increasing biodiversity, improving the water cycle, sequestering carbon and increasing resilience to climate change. Adopting philosophies including permaculture, biodynamics, grassfed (rather than grainfed) livestock and crop rotations amongst many others, eating food from regenerative producers improves human health and the health of the planet at large. And interestingly enough, it's the way longevity cultures have been feeding themselves and caring for the land for centuries.

▲ ▲ ▲

NUTRITION

It's Not All About Your Genes

Mimi Kirk (b. 1939) is my second favourite vegan behind John Robbins. Kirk has been voted the World's Sexiest Vegetarian over 50 (when she was 74) and has been a vegan since her early 30s. When Kirk joined me on *100 Not Out*, she was quick to warn against the danger of buying into the story of family genes.

"I'm the youngest of seven. My mother outlived four of her children," she told me. "My mum lived to be 95, but she was on a lot of prescription drugs. I have an 89-year old sister who takes 18 pills per day, and she's definitely fading. Both of my sisters have cancer. Parkinsons, diabetes and leukemia are in our family, as are high blood pressure, strokes, high cholesterol – everything you can imagine! A lot of these happened at an early age – and I've managed to keep these at bay. A lot of people say 'it's all about the genes'. Well, longevity might be about genes in some way, but some researchers say genes only contribute to 20% of our longevity. (In any case, life) isn't about living long, it's about living well. I might have the longevity gene, but not so much the healthy part of it, so that I have done on my own. I really feel I've manipulated that part so I don't have what my other family members have had."

If you grew up as Mimi Kirk did (in a family that doesn't support an exceptional diet), avoid buying into the belief that you are doomed to live a life of illness. Heed Kirk's example; if you decide to transform your diet, your genes will be in a more supportive environment to fully express their true potential.

Laying your future at the mercy of your genes is not only fatalistic, it robs you of taking any responsibility for your own health. Society will now accept almost any excuse for poor health, genes being one of them. *The Exceptionals*, meanwhile, have mastered the art of eating intelligently by linking their diet to what is most important to them.

The secret sauce is accountability

One of my major frustrations and curiosities in the early days of attending personal growth events was why so many people who attended did *nothing* with what they had just learned. They leave inspired and ready to make positive change in their life, only to fall off the bandwagon just minutes, hours or days later. For many, personal growth events are just like New Year's resolutions, just more expensive.

One example sticks out more than most. In 2007, Sarah and I attended a health retreat in Fiji, where we went on a juice cleanse. Very little food was consumed over the six days (with the support of health practitioners), replaced with loads of water and juice. The message towards the end of the event was on just how important the first 24 to 48 hours after the cleanse was, keeping in mind that the digestive system was not ready for large amounts of processed food.

The idea was to simply eat small amounts of natural foods, and slowly reintroduce more complex foods. So whilst sitting at the airport getting ready to fly home, what do we see? One of the attendees – let's call him Andrew – was licking his lips tucking in to a beer and meat pie!

Now just to be clear, I'm happy for Andrew to do whatever he wants! That is his human right. What I find intensely fascinating is that Andrew just spent a week of his life, $10,000, and possibly a week of unpaid leave attending an event to improve his body and mind, and whilst being told over and over and over again that the worst thing you could do after the event was to go back and start eating processed food, that's exactly what he did!

Now, why is that? Why did some people attend this event and allow it to be the springboard into an even more exceptional life, whilst others treated it as an expensive holiday in Fiji and then went back to the same life, same habits, and same behaviours?

The answer is accountability. During the cleanse, Andrew was accountable to the group and facilitators (and he had no available temptation).

As soon as we left though, Andrew had no one but himself to hold him accountable. His behaviour further demonstrated that he had not identified a reason strong enough to ensure he would behave in the recommended way. Would exceptional nutrition make him a better entrepreneur, father, partner, or friend? How would eating intelligently positively impact each area of his exceptional life? If he had asked these questions and truly owned the answers, I believe his behaviour would have been different.

Why the God of Sight quit smoking

Nepal's 'God of Sight', esteemed eye surgeon Dr Sanduk Ruit, used to spend the majority of his downtime with a cigarette in one hand and a stiff drink in the other. "You have a stupid excuse that you work so hard and you're so tired and you need something to relax you," Dr Ruit admitted to me on *100 Not Out*. "That's all bullshit I think. I really used to enjoy smoking, for a long time. First, I tried stopping smoking for a few intervals and never succeeded. Then what happened was, when my wife was eight months pregnant with my second child – we were in the bedroom just lying down and my wife was at my side and I lit up a cigarette and then my wife gave me a very nice soft dialogue, saying, 'It's OK. I can manage to smoke a little bit but do you want to also let your child inside me smoke too?' This really hit me very hard. I got up immediately and threw the cigarette away and decided that was it. If I want to live, this is the most important thing I can do. Without stopping it abruptly you can never stop it. My suggestion to everybody is you can't stop something in phases. That doesn't work. You have to find a good cause – either religious or family or whatever – and then, just stop it."

Not only did Dr Ruit quit smoking when he linked it to his role as a father and husband; he quit alcohol when he realised what impact it was having on his personal and professional life. His remarkable story has been captured in Ali Gripper's biography, *The Barefoot Surgeon*.

Exceptional Exercise 4.1:
Who or what keeps you accountable?

Do you have a cause or reason strong enough for you to improve what you eat, how you eat and who you eat with? If your reason for eating intelligently is only about you, exceptional nutrition is unlikely to be sustainable. So what is the *reason* or who is the *person or people* who keeps you accountable to hold high standards? To help you clarify your answer, I'll share with you my accountabilities around food. Each day, in order for me to do what I love and maintain high standards in all eight areas of life, eating energising and high quality food is essential. Eating well keeps my mind sharp and my motivation high during my working hours. It allows me to be present with family and friends and simply helps me to be the best version of myself.

Secondly, in my current phase of life, I know my children are watching me and observing almost every morsel of food that passes my lips! If I eat something they are not familiar with or that they *know* is not healthy, I better have a good reason! I don't want to teach them one thing, and do another. I believe the most disempowering message a parent or leader could ever teach a child is 'do as I say, not as I do'. I make almost every decision in my personal and professional life as if my children are watching. They don't have to understand it in the moment (they may be too young), but as long as I can congruently explain my actions to them, I am at peace.

Refuse to let poor nutrition infect your exceptional life

When you consider the real cost of a poor diet – life – and the mess it creates for you and the people around you, every meal you eat takes on an entirely new meaning. The first consequence that shows up is dis-ease.

A lack of ease throughout your daily life manifests in the form of fatigue, brain fog, poor moods, lack of will and many more quiet clues. These symptoms are providing whispering feedback that mediocrity exists. We feel it, and often we ignore it and carry on. As long as one focuses on surviving over thriving, mediocrity exists and so does its consequences.

Over time, in the spirit of gradual accumulation, acute dis-ease slowly but surely graduates to chronic disease. A few extra kilos turns into 20; overweight turns into obesity; years of poor eating and digestive complaints develop into diabetes or cancer. There's no mistaking it; just as most dis-ease was created by mediocre standards and decisions, 40% of many cancers and 44% of diabetes are the result of years of mediocre decisions, made one 'harmless, everything in moderation' meal at a time.

These conditions aren't just a disease of the body, they become a disease of life. Disease stops people working and can cause premature retirement, which may lead to depression and other forms of mental illness. Disease makes movement impossible or far more difficult, resulting in more diseases including dementia. Disease impacts your social and family life, often in the form of loneliness and emotional distance. Disease impacts your ability to travel and prevents the freedom to experience your life's dreams. Disease costs money and creates emotional turmoil and financial havoc. Disease can be the spirit maker for some, yet for many it is the spirit breaker, leading to a premature, heart-breaking death.

On water

I'm yet to find water filters sitting pride of place in the kitchen of many graceful agers. They tend to drink tap water, and that in itself is the exceptional behaviour, given that many people born in the first half of the 20th century grew up being taught water was only to shower in and pour over the garden or a teabag. At the other extreme, I know others who won't drink water in public and will only consume it if it's spring water or put through a reverse osmosis system.

I'm not one to drink water out of a tap too often, but if I'm travelling (which I do regularly), I'm not going to panic at the thought of having tap water. I'm also conscious not to buy multiple single use plastic water bottles throughout my travels. What's clear is that, at the very least, quality water consumption is a great insurance policy. Apart from an additional cost (which, over the life of the filter is negligible), there is nothing to lose from having a water filter. I'd rather have my fair share of quality water than not have it.

According to the *Journal of Biological Chemistry*, the adult human body is between 55 and 60% water. Our heart and brain are 73% water, our lungs are 83% water and even our bones are 31% water.[12] These numbers alone demonstrate a diet rich in water is a good idea. This doesn't have to be from drinking water only. Eating water rich foods (many fruits and salad vegetables) will benefit hydration and optimal body function. Longevity cultures have a rich tradition of drinking tea, be it herbal, green or some other variety. However you take it, just drink water.

How much water should you drink?

8 glasses or two litres per day somehow became the standard measure across the western world for many health authorities. Yet a 100kg elite athlete will surely need more water than a 13-year old teenager. In addition, water intake will vary based on the climate you live in, your physical activity levels, and your gender.

Whilst still limited, consumption based on body size is a far more individual and undoubtedly more accurate measure. Your ideal water intake is likely to be 25–35ml for every kilogram of bodyweight. For me (73kg), that works out at 1.83 to 2.55 litres per day. Keep in mind that tea and coffee are diuretics, so it's important to drink two glasses of water for every caffeinated drink. Herbal tea, on the other hand, can count towards your intake.

On alcohol

Longevity cultures and *The Exceptionals* – from Holocaust surivivors to everyday centenarians – are quite fond of having a small amount of alcohol. Whilst there is no doubt that some people fare better on abstinence over moderation, the majority of *Exceptionals* I have come across enjoy a drink. The drinking culture on the little Greek island of Ikaria is one I think best reflects not only the purpose of alcohol, but a great respect for it's power to build up and equally destroy.

Ikaria's Five Golden Rules of Alcohol

1. **Eat when you drink** – it will allow you to eat more and drink more over the long run.
2. **Never drink on an empty stomach.** Many Western cultures say "eating is cheating", however in Ikaria nothing could be further from the truth. Upon arrival at a panigiri, Ikarians drink goat broth to line their stomachs in preparation for what can be a 14-hour festival.
3. **Getting drunk is frowned upon.** Getting tipsy however, is seen as a great social lubricant.
4. Ikarians only **drink in the company of others** and never alone. Alcohol is not seen as a coping mechanism for when times are tough – that's what friends and family are for.
5. And finally, Ikarians drink their own wine or the wine of their neighbours. They **know where the wine came from**, and whilst the wine may not be certified organic, it's homegrown, likely biodynamic, sprayfree and made with love. If they're not sure what to expect, locals will bring their own wine to a social function, such is their focus on quality over quantity.

On veganism

"Veganism can be scientifically and successfully accomplished," Dr John Demartini shared with me on *100 Not Out*. "But it does require thought and planning and understanding of nutrients. I've seen some people who have gone vegan for a long period of time who start having skin conditions, bone conditions and bowel conditions. They become so sensitive and emotionally charged against food that if they even get around those other foods they get sick, so I've seen extremes lead to disturbances. I'm a firm believer there's a value in moderation, and the diversity of foods to make sure that the adequate nutrients are met and I think we are designed for the adaptability for all of the foods. Excessive proteins, excessive meats, excessive fats, excessive sugars, excessive anything usually has its toll. It's just like putting all of your money into one investment. That's usually unwise. It's wise to have a little bit of a diversity," he says.

Demartini's conclusion? "I can't say that I know a lot of vegans that have done it for 60, 70, or 80 years. And I can't say that a lot of them don't sneak other foods in. But I know that scientifically it can be done. It's just very impractical for daily life for most people. So I'm a firm believer to allow yourself the variety of foods your body has all types of teeth for, all types of digestion and chewing and swallowing. It's meant to have a variety of food."

As a former vegan I can heavily relate to a lot of Dr Demartini's words. I ended my vegan diet after six years of dedicated plant-based eating. Here's what I discovered: being vegan for a week, a month or a year will bring fabulous results for the individual. You'll lose weight, your skin may clear, your energy may soar and, if you listen to enough vegans, you'll be on the shortcut to enlightenment. I'm not exaggerating – that's exactly what I believed. On reflection though, I was anything but enlightened, in fact I was looking down upon my poor misinformed meat-eaters from my judgemental vegan high horse.

In reality, my vegan diet had yielded similar results to most diets; an increase in energy, some weight loss and then a plateau. My weight plateaued at 73kg after six months as a vegan and has been there ever since, even though I now consume meat and small amounts of dairy and alcohol.

What I have come to learn is that not a tribe or culture exists today or ever did who subsisted on a 100% plant-based diet and enjoyed quality *and* quantity of life. Loma Linda, California, is considered the plant-based Blue Zone, yet only 4% of their Seventh Day Adventist population is strictly vegan. I'm yet to find a centenarian vegan to interview on *100 Not Out* who has been a vegan since the day they were born. At the time of print, my view is that there is not a single person on the planet who has been a vegan for 100 years. If you find one, please send me their contact details as I would love to interview them!

▲ ▲ ▲

How to Eat and Who to Eat With

It's incredibly easy to get stuck in the vacuum of focusing solely on what to eat. Decoding the matrix of proteins, carbohydrates and fats however, is not the answer to eating intelligently. Learning *how* to eat, and making an effort to eat in the company of others, is perhaps just as, if not more important than the food that passes your lips.

Eat at the table

In 2019, more than 130 million Americans consumed frozen dinners (also known as TV dinners).[13] The name TV dinner was created in 1953 by the inventor of the meal, Gerry Thomas, when owning a television became a status symbol. Today, the rise of television has led to the decline and potential extinction of the traditional family dinner. Whilst it's unlikely these figures will reverse, a sneak peek in to the lives of the *Exceptionals* will show that they are yet to receive the memo encouraging them to embrace TV dinners.

The humble dining table provides us with the opportunity to let off steam from the day, connect with family and friends, learn about what's happening in their lives, and on a grander scale, share our vulnerabilities, fears and concerns about anything troubling us. There is perhaps no greater mental health first aid than a dining table, great food and the company of empowering human beings.

Eat with others

Food was never meant to be exclusively a solo experience. Whilst many of us choose to live alone, part of the magic of food is its ability to bring people together. Statistically, we eat 50% of our main meals and 70% of our snacks alone.[14] Couple this with the TV dinner figures and our global dining lifestyle is beginning to look somewhat deplorable. And whilst I have no problem with eating snacks alone, my concern is that when we *do* eat together, it's in front of the TV or with our phones by our side.

If you know you are a statistic of modern dining, simply start with one main meal you would like to eat with others. Food eaten alongside people you love can stimulate quality conversation, from sharing victories and challenges from the day to deeper questions about life. If you live alone, you can invite a friend(s) or family over once or twice per week for dinner in order to add some variety and social stimulation to your life. You may even organise with a friend to alternate midweek dinners. In addition, I know people who travel to all four corners of the globe and will sit down to breakfast whilst FaceTiming their family who are enjoying dinner. They are both eating at the dining table, 'virtually' in the company of others, and engaging in conversation.

However you choose to do this, when you eat with others you are likely to –

- ➢ Take more pride in the meal you prepare
- ➢ Chew your food and eat more slowly (because there's a conversation to be had)
- ➢ Make the dining experience last longer, allowing you to relax
- ➢ Improve digestion

Chew like you mean it

Eating alone and on the run is not the only casualty from an increase in the speed of daily life. Another is the speed of which we eat – or the time we allot to meal times. Busy-ness is akin to a metastatic disease, slowly taking over multiple parts of our life. Breakfast *never* used to be a car-ride meal. Now it's the only way many people have it. Dinner was *never* a TV meal; now it's the usual setup for many families. How can we possibly enjoy our meals *together* when we only give ourselves five minutes, if that, to enjoy it?

Whilst many people chew between five and 10 times for each mouthful, an exceptional standard is to reach at least 20. The most common resistance I get from others is the 'disgusting' feeling of having small fragments of food in one's mouth. Seriously, think about this for a moment. This is *exactly* what your teeth are designed to do! Not only that, the act of chewing stimulates digestion, so that by the time your masticated food reaches your large and small intestines, they can more effortlessly extract the nutrients your body requires without working overtime on breaking the food down. As a result, your energy soars (blood isn't being rushed to your stomach for the digestive overload), your toilet experiences become far more pleasant, indigestion can become a thing of the past and your dining experience is enriched.

> **Exceptional Exercise 4.2: Count your chews**
>
> For such a small, simple, and free practice, chewing can have an incredible impact on you socially, physically, mentally and emotionally. Give it a go by counting your chews at your next meal and increasing by at least one with each mouthful. As my dentist says, "chew like you mean it", and enjoy the positive consequences.

Breathe

I typically arrive at the dining table in an adrenalised state. I've just made breakfast for the family, am in the middle of a busy work day, or scrambling to close up the day amid a raucous banging on my office door from my enthusiastic children. The result is that I'm in a state of stress when I take my seat, and it takes a little while for the body and mind to calm down and adjust.

The Exceptionals who live with a faith or belief in a higher power have a ritual of giving thanks for their meal before eating. When our family gives a blessing of gratitude for the meal that we have before us I notice my heart rate drop, my body relax and switch gears to the ritual of eating rather than working.

> ### Exceptional Exercise 4.3: The art of deep breathing
>
> The simple ritual of taking some deep breaths before eating will do wonders for your body, mind and soul. Many forms of deep breathing have become popular, almost to the point of overwhelm. The key to deep breathing is to work on the breath coming from the diaphragm or stomach rather than the chest and shoulders. This can be a work in progress, depending on your stress levels. I like to take 10 deep breaths before meals in a ratio of 1:1:1, where the numbers represent breathing in, holding, and breathing out. For example, I will regularly take 10 deep breaths: breathing in for seven seconds, holding for seven, and exhaling for seven.

Serve your meals family style

Many cultures do this out of habit, and many of us have done it on special occasions when feeding a large group of friends or family. Serving the meal 'family style', where the food is served on platters or large plates rather than on each individual plate, is littered with small, but meaningful benefits, including –

- Asking for food to be passed around the table stimulates conversation and improves social skills (for adults and children alike).
- Whilst some believe family style encourages overeating, the opposite in fact is true. Family style encourages us to be considerate of others, meaning you'll likely take smaller portions so that each person at the table will get their fair share.
- Family style provides children with a fabulous level of control. Children choose food that *their* body wants rather than what the parent or carer wants them to have. This is a big challenge for many parents, however if the meal is nutritious there is no problem in your child having more protein one night, and more carbohydrates the next.
- Family style encourages children to learn the art of patience. Learning that our needs aren't always instantly met is an incredible life lesson.

This is not to suggest that all meals need to be served family style in order for the above benefits to manifest. Breakfast and lunch in our family home is often served individually, whereas the dinner is often served family style.

Stop eating before you're full

Ayurvedic nutrition has an eating philosophy dating back to the 4th century BC that: 'You should fill one third of the stomach with liquid, another third with food, and leave the rest empty'. Traditional Chinese Medicine declares *chi fan qi fen bao, san fen han* which translates to eating until you are 70 per cent full. As mentioned earlier, the Okinawans have an eating philosophy derived from Confucious – *hara hachi bu* – or 'eat until you are eight parts (out of ten) full'. One culture (Japan) sits atop the longevity ladder, whilst the other two (India and China) represent more than 25% of the global population.

Stopping to eat before you feel full is not a modern fad or biohack to improve your quality and quantity of life; it is a practice steeped in the history of humanity that protects, respects and lengthens life.

Mind your own plate

I grew up being constantly reminded by my parents to stop sniggering at what my sisters did or didn't eat and to instead "mind your own plate". My sister, Olivia, has never had a wild appetite, and I remember constantly making fun of her or scrambling to peck at her leftovers. It seems many in society were never taught to mind their own plate, and instead they judge, berate and condescend others for their own dietary choices. Whilst you may find it difficult to stop caring what others eat, the least you can do as an *Exceptional* is to love your fellow eaters for who they are – men, women and children of the world – instead of what they do or don't eat. All of us are going on our own journey of self-discovery, where the path is unique with various speeds and bumps along the way. What we eat, the way we eat, who we eat with, and why we eat, have very strong links to our childhood, which no one else has lived. We can never fully know what it's like to walk in someone else's shoes.

> ### The vegan, the carnivore and the chicken lover
> Nutritionist Cyndi O'Meara reminds me of a female Bear Grylls; a strong, lean, hunter-gatherer, get-your-hands-dirty organ-and-offal devouring meat-eater. I'm embellishing but you get the picture. Carren Smith is a Bali-bomb-surviving keynote speaker who couldn't kill a mosquito even if it was sucking the last drop of blood out of her body. Carren is a dedicated vegan. Kim Morrison is a self-love guru who will dry retch at the idea of bone marrow. She eats white meat – chicken and fish – but cannot comprehend eating red meat. Cyndi, Kim and Carren are best friends. They met through serendipity and have gone through the highs and lows of life with each other for over a decade. The vegan, the carnivore and the dry-retching chicken lover never entertained the idea of ending a friendship based on dietary choices or food philosophy. They simply love each other for who they are, not what they eat.

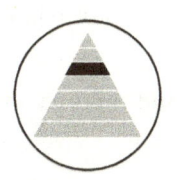

FAMILY

*"I don't know that it exists, the perfect family.
It's always complicated."*
– Ben Mendelsohn

The notion that *family comes first* is both fraught with danger and holds the secret to a great quality of life. To overindulge in family, like good food, is a recipe for unmet expectations and unfulfilled dreams. To ignore and devalue family is the recipe for bitter and twisted relationships and terrible self-esteem. Striking the right balance between family and the rest of your exceptional life is equal parts delicate and essential.

The Exceptionals acknowledge that family is complicated and shun attempts to simplify it, knowing that such work is futile. There are up to 10 relationships that can impact us – grandparents, parents, siblings, children, grandchildren, intimate partners, cousins, aunties and uncles, in-laws and steps. And I haven't even mentioned adopted, orphaned or foster families.

The power of exceptional family relationships stretches far beyond emotional connection. There is a disturbing link between the quality of some family relationships – namely your parents and your intimate partner – and your physical health. Lifelong smokers go close to outliving divorced non-smokers[1] whilst cold and tolerant relationships with parents can be a recipe for a mid-life medical crisis.[2]

On the flipside, marriage and children are not the cure-all for longevity. Look to any centenarian Holocaust survivor or war widow and you'll see that family and longevity do not hold hands. Many an *Exceptional* has buried children and their soul mate. What an exceptional family life will do is exponentially improve the quality of your life. Your birthdays are celebrated with loved ones, Christmas Day is bereft of awkward or heated exchanges, family holidays are enjoyed rather than filled with narkiness and your regular social gatherings are cherished rather than dreaded.

▲ ▲ ▲

The True Meaning and Purpose of Family

Trevor Hendy AM (b. 1968) is a national icon in Australia. A six-time Ironman champion and member of the Australian Sport Hall Of Fame, Hendy had the epitome of what many people would call the 'perfect life', with success, fame, marriage, two children, a big house and a luxurious lifestyle ticked off.

Unbeknownst to many though, Hendy and wife Jacki were struggling in their marriage, and after seven years and two children, Kristelle and TJ, the two separated. Hendy went on to marry his second wife, Jo, and have two children together, Bailey and Jaali. To this day, Hendy and Jacki remain close friends.

"I was talking at a networking breakfast that Jacki organises," Hendy recounted on an interview of *100 Not Out*. "Jo was there and Jacki was there – we're one big extended family. We've been through all sorts of ups and downs together but there's a lot of love and care and a real sort of brotherly-sisterly connection between all of us. The audience were blown away that we were all there together at this event. You know – there's my first wife there and there's my second wife and there's the four kids and we're all in the one room. And this created a conversation in the room, so my keynote turned into a facilitated talk as to how we make our family work."

Hendy went on to say: "Someone stood up and told the story of a Chinese emperor whose townspeople had prepared this incredible pot and they come to present it to him on his visit to the city and they (accidentally) drop it and it smashes into one thousand pieces. Everybody's horrified and this emperor, who everybody loved and was very wise, said 'Stop! Don't touch it. Just bring all the pieces back together.' He had them glue all the pieces back together in whatever way they fell, and then he put this huge mosaic (containing the pieces of the broken pot) up on the wall, and he said to the townspeople, 'Isn't that far more beautiful than the original pot?' I literally cried on stage, standing there with the broken pieces of my life, and said 'Wow. What we have now is more beautiful than what we would have had had I gone down this path of white picket fences, cars, houses, mortgage, and everything else.' I was always destined to have a 'mess' so that I could have a really beautiful mess at the end of it, which came together in very organic ways."

You may not have a family life quite like Hendy's. In fact, yours may be far *more* complicated and messy. I'm tipping you've had a seemingly beautiful pot fall to the ground and smash into a thousand pieces. Your family has fragmented in some way – childhood trauma, unapproved marriage, clashing in-laws, divorce, death, estrangement, violence, bankruptcy, crime, deception, disease – are all examples of pots smashing to the ground.

The difference between average and exceptional relationships is how the pieces are put back together. Depending on the circumstances, many people believe the broken pot should be put back in a way so that 'things were like they used to be'. At the other extreme, for many the broken pot represents a deed that is irreconcilable and unforgivable. *The Exceptionals*, like the emperor, decide to create a mosaic with the same pieces of life, crafting in the process an entirely new life that wouldn't be possible without the pot smashing in the first place. They put the pieces back together, acknowledging that things can never be like they were, but that life can be even more beautiful with a new constellation of life events.

The decision to make in this section of your exceptional life is whether you choose to place a limit on what's possible for your family relationships. If you choose to leave the broken pot on the floor, and continue to do so as more pots fall to the floor as life unfolds, there is really only one end. And that's an ugly combination of bitterness, hate, pessimism, cynicism, loneliness, regret and despair.

Nothing is more reflective of the broken pot scattered on the floor than a lonely soul, sitting in a nursing home for years on end because no one in the family cares enough to visit. Weeks, months, and years pass by without a visit from children, a spouse or even friends because multiple smashed pots have never been rebuilt into mosaics. Please don't let this nightmare become your all too common reality.

> *"I love and adore them all and can say I've looked at the clouds from both sides now."*
> *– Trevor Hendy*

Finding function in the dysfunctional family

Did you grow up in a 'perfect' family? A family where everyone got along all of the time and you had no major challenges? My research suggests there isn't a single soul that has experienced an all-pleasure no-pain family life.

Instead, tough times, dysfunction and unconditional love share a special bond. Millions of marriages were born out of the war, giving rise to the Baby Boomer generation. The strength of a family unit is often defined by heartache, be it a health crisis, family death, divorce, business upheaval or some other form of challenge.

If my parents had a sensational marriage that lasted the test of time, there's every chance I wouldn't be the dedicated husband I am today. During my childhood, Dad worked long hours as a newsagent and struggled to prioritise quality time with my mum. Like many marriages,

Mum and Dad had different views and values on time and money — differences that eventually led to their separation when I was 10. As a result, whilst our home life wasn't traumatic, my childhood memories aren't filled with delightful, connected family time that included my sisters and both parents. Over the years, what I have come to realise more than anything is my parents taught me how marriage should not be. I have constantly worked at having the opposite marriage of my parents; a lesson I am grateful to both my mum and dad for.

One of my worst family nightmares is facing the reality my dad did: reversing out of the driveway, no longer the homeowner and dweller of the quarter-acre memory maker he'd designed and help build; the place where childhood memories were made to last a lifetime; the place that would be the centre of many conversations for years to come. He wouldn't be part of the family home memory bank; he wouldn't be in the photos swimming in the pool or at the dinner table blowing out a birthday cake. Instead, 15 years of marriage would end with my dad sleeping on a single mattress on the floor of my grandmother's spare room.

My dad idolised his mum, Alma. I never met Dad's father, Earle Pearce. Earle died at 52 after a long battle with alcoholism. My dad, 21 at the time, arrived home from work one night and found Earle dead in his bed. "Good" was the word Dad muttered upon finding my grandfather, relieved that a childhood filled with stress and tension had come to its end. Dad left Earle in bed, slept more soundly than he had in years, and revealed the news to my grandma the next morning.

"I was relieved for Mum that she didn't have to deal with Dad anymore, but she was distraught," recalls Dad. "Dad wasn't abusive, he was just a drunk. I'd be dropped off by the school bus and see my dad sprawled on the garden out the front. One day, he drove his car through the fence of the front yard."

The example my grandfather set was incredibly influential. My dad's three siblings all grew up to be heavy drinkers and smokers in their adult years. All three have sadly passed away, aged 66, 74 and 80. My dad, so appalled at the example his father set, has approached his life very differently to his siblings in relation to alcohol. Dad rarely drinks and doesn't smoke and when asked why, his response is, "If you met my father, you'd know why." In a mind-bending twist of the genetic knife, I believe my aunties Helen and Margaret, and uncle Doug would also explain their own lifestyle with the same answer.

It's time to redefine what love is

Was my grandfather a bad dad? Did he wreck his children's lives and that of my grandmother? Whilst I think it's easy to say that he did, a broader view demonstrates that he taught his children some powerful lessons in perhaps unorthodox ways. My dad says home life made it difficult to complete homework and be fully engaged in his education. As a result, Dad never finished high school and instead took a job at supermarket chain Coles, where he went on to complete an executive program. Dad had a knack for selling and spent time buying, growing and selling newsagencies before carving out a career at the media company News Limited.

It's quite plausible to suggest that Earle's absence as a father had a powerful impact on my dad's business success and family life. Dad financed our private school education by delivering newspapers early each weekday, and on weekends he would spoil us and take us on regular trips to the MCG to watch our beloved Melbourne Football Club. Whilst Dad was arguably overcommitted to his career, he always found a way to spend quality time with his children. I wonder if that would have been the case if Earle had been a 'better' dad.

Learning to appreciate the differences in family members

As you navigate through this section and the tricky maze of family dynamics, what becomes clear is just how different each member of the family is. What you want for your life (in each of the eight areas) is going to be different to what your parents, siblings, partner or children want in theirs. My wish is that you truly own how unfulfilling family life would be if we were all similar and wanted the same kind of life.

This section invites you to master five key family dynamics (the ones that apply) – your parents, grandparents, siblings, partner and children. I have given each relationship a theme, which can be applied to any other. The theme of parents is forgiveness and for grandparents the focus is exemplification. Connection and touch is the theme of sibling relationships, whilst acceptance is the message of intimate relationships. With children, the focus is on unconditional love. All of these themes apply to every relationship you have.

> *"Feelings of worth can flourish only in an atmosphere where individual differences are appreciated, mistakes are tolerated, communication is open, and rules are flexible – the kind of atmosphere that is found in a nurturing family."*
> **– Virginia Satir**

▲ ▲ ▲

Relationship 1: Parents

One of the most alarming studies I've ever come across is a Harvard University study asking 125 undergraduate students to rate their relationship with their parents.[3] Admittedly, it was only done on 125 people, yet I've shared this study with thousands of people at events and the nods of the head and the hands raised are in accordance with the following findings.

The students were asked to rank their relationship with their parents as one of these four options – very close, warm and friendly, tolerant, or strained and cold.

35 years later the study came to life. 91% of the people who had a tolerant or strained and cold relationship with their mother had suffered a serious medical crisis by their mid 50s.[4] The definition of medical crisis is not finite, but it includes coronary artery disease, high blood pressure, ulcers, and alcoholism.

These people had twice the risk of experiencing a medical crisis than those who had a warm and friendly or very close relationship with their mother (45%).[5] On the paternal side, 82% of the people who had a tolerant or strained and cold relationship with their father had suffered a serious medical crisis by their mid 50s.[6] And incredibly, 100% of the people who had a tolerant or strained and cold relationship with both parents had suffered a serious medical crisis by their mid 50s.[7]

So the two most important questions to ask right now are:
How would you rank the relationship with your mother?
How would you rank the relationship with your father?

How to improve your relationship with your parents

If you've answered those two questions and have a tolerant or strained and cold relationship with one or both parents, the most important decision to make is how you intend to improve it to very close or warm and friendly. As we age, we begin to realise that our parents were adult human beings attempting to work out their own lives and often were not aware of our expectations or how to meet them. For many of us, adulthood brings with it the realisation our parents are not the heroes we thought they were when we were young.

If you resist the decision to improve your relationships, the Harvard research (and my anecdotal findings in sharing this with thousands of people) suggests your health in mid-life is at risk. There is only one path to graduating from tolerant or strained relationships to very close and warm, and that is to take the road less travelled of forgiveness.

Forgiveness

Forgiveness is arguably the most difficult step you can take in progressing your life. Some may argue self-love is more challenging, however a major part of loving ourselves is accepting and owning all the parts of who we are – a process which requires forgiveness.

Forgiveness is challenging because at the source of everything to forgive is a human being – you and/or others – and these people live in your daily life or in your memories. If memories could be deleted, forgive and forget may be more appropriate, but given that's not the case, forgiving in spite of *not* forgetting is true forgiveness. You might forgive your mum for having an affair and then the next day you listen to her whinge and moan about her new partner! These moments are not random, annoying events but instead are perfectly placed mini challenges to test the true resolve and authenticity of your forgiveness. As a result, this is not something you can do once and tick it off your list. People and events often require being forgiven over and over and over again, and it's for this reason that society honours the likes of Nelson Mandela, Malala Yousafzai and *The Exceptionals* who live with unconditional love in their heart.

You don't need to experience 27 years of improper imprisonment to be exceptional in the art of forgiveness, but you do need to buck the trend of what many people see as forgiveness. The *Oxford Dictionary* says forgiving is to "stop feeling angry or resentful towards someone for an offence, flaw or mistake". But to *stop* or *remove* an emotion only creates space for a new emotion to take its place. If you're not thorough in the way you forgive, you may find yourself replacing your resentment with indifference or repression, which is nothing more than a subdued version of your anger, resentment or hatred of that person. That is not forgiveness; it is a smaller dose of the same toxic disease. Authentic forgiveness is not about condoning or excusing people's behaviour; true forgiveness is coming from a place of compassion for the individual and gratitude that these events have actually occurred in your life. That doesn't mean that you *wanted* them to happen; it means that you have accepted *that* they happened, even if you're not sure *why* they happened. Genocide and murder are perhaps two of the more commonly 'unforgiveable' acts, so let's go straight for the jugular and see how it's done.

The Holocaust survivor who forgave Hitler

During the Nazi invasion of Prague in 1940, Alice Herz-Sommer's family fled to Palestine in seek of refuge. Alice remained in Prague with her mother, Sofie, who was not fit enough to travel. The inevitable happened, with Alice, Sofie, Alice's husband Leopold and their son, Raphael eventually arrested. Sofie, 72, was murdered shortly after their arrest, whilst Leopold, Alice and Raphael were held at the Theresienstadt concentration camp. Leopold was later transferred to Dachau and died there from typhus just six weeks before the liberation.

What makes the story of Alice Herz-Sommer particularly remarkable is her ability to forgive Adolf Hitler and the Nazis for the trauma inflicted on her family and the Jewish community.

One of the more repeated questions of Alice during interviews was about Hitler, something along the lines of: "Alice, surely you hate Hitler for what he did to you, your family, and your fellow Jews?" Her answer was always similar: "I never hate…hate begets hate…hatred eats the soul of the hater, not the hated…I have no room for pessimism or hate."[8]

Reread that mantra. *I have no room for pessimism or hate.* Do you have room for pessimisim or hatred in your life? Consider just how socially acceptable it is for us to be outraged, pessimistic and hateful towards others these days and you'll get a glimpse of just how exceptional Alice Herz-Sommer really was.

Herz-Sommer refused to let Hitler impact the rest of her life. Whilst she acknowledged the atrocities of what had occurred in her life, she refused to give them power and make them part of her script for the future. By the way she spoke and in her official biography *A Century Of Wisdom*, one can only feel that Alice chose to be grateful for the test of her spirit. Alice Herz-Sommer lived to be 110 and was the oldest female survivor of the Holocaust at the time of her death.

To go through her experiences and live her life in this way is not just a beacon of light for all of us, it goes to show just how limitless our potential as human beings really is. "I look at the good," Alice said. "When you are relaxed, your body is always relaxed. When you are pessimistic, your body behaves in an unnatural way. It is up to us whether we look at the good or the bad."

If one can go through the Holocaust and still live with a remarkable level of grace, surely you and I can lose any 'stinking thinking' about life or other people, and begin to become more accepting and unconditional towards others.

The father who forgave the murderer of his daughter

Gary Ridgway is known as the 'Green River Killer'. He is currently serving a life sentence in the Washington State Penitentiary. He was convicted for the murder and rape of 49 women between 1982 and 1998, the second most prolific serial killer in United States history according to confirmed murders. Before being sentenced, family members of the victims were given the opportunity to say their final words to Ridgway. It was one of the most dramatic and heart-wrenching courtroom scenes you're likely to see. Here are three statements from relatives of the victims.

"He's an animal. I wish for him to have a long, suffering, cruel death!"[9]

Vicky Ware *(sister of Kelly Ware)*

"He's going to go to hell, and that's where he belongs!"[10]

Carol Estes *(mother of Debra Estes)*

"There are people here who hate you; I'm not one of them. You've made it difficult for me to live up to what I believe, but that is what God says to do. That's to forgive. You are forgiven, sir."[11]

Robert Rule *(father of Linda Rule)*

How did someone like Robert Rule arrive at that level of forgiveness? Rule was deeply religious and his response is an inspirational example of the muscle of forgiveness being exercised. Most of us refuse to exercise the forgiveness muscle, and therefore it atrophies as we get older (have you ever noticed how quickly children forgive?).

As a result of this atrophy, we all have a different threshold or set of rules when it comes to forgiveness. Some won't forgive a person for being late to a meeting, whilst others will forgive the murderer of their child. People like Alice Herz-Sommer and Robert Rule seem to have no threshold. Not only did they live with truly unconditional love, they embody what I like to call *limitless souls*. As hard as it is, whatever occurred in their life was not worth holding on to. We are all limitless souls, and it's through the act of forgiveness that we begin to believe it and see it shine through.

Don't forgive and forget

Forgetting is as good as turning a blind eye or the other cheek to what's occurred that causes so much unrest in the first place. "Forgiveness doesn't mean forget what happened," according to His Holiness the Dalai Lama (b. 1935). "Practising forgiveness does not mean accepting wrong doing." Instead, the Dalai Lama contends that forgiveness allows you "to not let the behaviour of others destroy your inner peace".

In practical terms, forgiving *and* forgetting completely changes the dynamic of the relationship you have with the person. An elephant in the room forever remains in the psyche of everyone affected. And you can be sure that the topic *never* comes up in conversation, because 'we don't talk about *that* now'. When you forgive and do *not* forget, you are showing a far stronger form of love. You're saying, "I acknowledge what happened and I not only forgive you, I have compassion for you and your behaviour." That is the exceptional, more difficult action, and the one with far more empowering consequences than holding on to hatred.

> *"Holding on to anger is like drinking poison and expecting the other person to die."*
> *– Unknown*

How strong is your forgiveness muscle?

How easily do you forgive? Is there a threshold where you find something unforgiveable? Do you hold on to injustice? Is infidelity unforgiveable? Is murder unforgiveable? What about mass murder? Where does it end? If someone in your family were murdered, would you forgive the perpetrator? Granted, these are massive hypothetical questions. If we talk about *unconditional* love, we are talking about a love *without* conditions. That means love transcends all crimes and despicable acts. Nelson Mandela, Robert Rule and Alice Herz-Sommer are examples of what unconditional love looks like in human form.

Forgiveness requires time and compassion

"It is strange in me that after some years I forgive them," Ada Murkies (b. 1922) told me on *100 Not Out* when asked about the Russians who murdered her father, Stefan, and 22,000 Polish military officers in the 1940 Katyn Forest Massacre. "If you don't forgive and constantly think about the cruelty they did, you can't start your happy life. That's why you need to forgive. You need to hope that life should be better."

Murkies leaves a clue in her answers as to the first pillar of forgiveness, and that is the passage of time. You are not expected to forgive minutes or hours after a traumatic event or ending of a toxic relationship. For many, authentic forgiveness is years in the making. At some point, *The Exceptionals* become acutely aware that hate doesn't serve anyone, except adding more fuel to the fire of resentment. To forgive, one must be willing to remove hate and replace it with the second pillar of forgiveness, which is compassion.

"We believe that hate is a disease," says Holocaust survivor, Eddie Jaku. "It's put in to you and you spread it and it becomes more and more. Hate inspires violence. Hate grows to such an extent that two or three people together become violent and kill somebody. This has to be eradicated and it has to be eradicated at home. Education doesn't start at school; it begins at home. I can assure you, I can speak on this until I am blue in my face. If the parents say, 'I hate Jews', the children will say, 'I hate Jews'. When I have a group of children or students here, I tell them 'promise me don't use this word hate from today'. That's important to me, to the world, to humanity."

How to forgive

There are a number of ways to forgive and the list below is by no means exhaustive. They exist to spur you into action on deciding *who* you choose to begin the forgiveness process with and *how* you want to do it. Here are five ways to forgive:

Forgiveness in writing

Writing a forgiveness letter is my favourite way to forgive someone. It can be used for someone dead or alive, local or non-local. It's a ferocious, aggressive, emotionally and spiritually cleansing process that can be full of tears and eventual joy and gratitude. The power of the letter is that it can be used in the other methods listed below. There are many forgiveness letter templates publicly available. Go to **marcuspearce.com.au/yourexceptionallife** to access the one I use personally and with clients.

You don't have to send your letter to the individual. Just the act of releasing the words of forgiveness and acknowledging your hurt is a way to help you towards healing. In fact, sometimes it helps to write your letter, then let it sit for a few weeks.

Forgiveness in person

This one is not for the faint-hearted. My suggestion is that you write a forgiveness letter first and then read it to the person when you are in their company.

Forgiveness over the phone

You might be in another state or country to the person you are forgiving. In this case I recommend reading your forgiveness letter to the person over the phone. Please give them warning of what is to come though!

Forgiveness through prayer or meditation

My personal view is that this method fulfils half the requirement to completely forgive. Robert Rule was a very religious man. I have no doubt that he prayed and prayed and prayed as he worked to forgive Gary Ridgway. The completion of the forgiveness, though, occurred in the courtroom. It would have been no use to pray day and night only to buckle when confronted with the killer in person. Moreover, Rule would have needed to practise forgiveness each time he felt the pain of loss and wave of grief for his daughter Linda.

Forgiveness through changed perspective

There is also the view that perhaps in actuality there is nothing to forgive. The work of Brené Brown, Byron Katie and Dr John Demartini will help you see the blessings and benefits of the event or person that you have hate and anger towards. "Forgiveness is not forgetting or walking away from accountability or condoning a hurtful act," says Brown. "It's the process of taking back and healing our lives so we can truly live."

Whether it is murder, rape, genocide, abuse, deception or loss of any kind, Dr Demartini has an unshakeable belief that they are all blessings in disguise. "I'm not a promoter of victim thinking," Dr Demartini told me on *100 Not Out*. "I'm a believer that we have control over our perceptions, decisions and actions and it's never what happens to us, it's how we perceive it. I'm interested in people taking whatever happens in life and using it to their greatest advantage so that they can do something extraordinary with their lives. The more challenges you've been through the more power you have access to."

Accepting the apology you'll never get

You may be reading this and wanting to forgive someone who has died or you are unlikely to ever see again in your life. If they're alive, they might be someone who will avoid your calls or refuse to open the door. According to writer Robert Brault, "Life becomes easier when you learn to accept the apology you never got." Don't expect people to apologise to you as a result of forgiving them. Instead, your job as an *Exceptional* is to show leadership by forgiving them without seeking an apology in return. Write the letter and read it out loud to the deceased person or estranged partner. You may even wish to visit their grave, pull out a photo or video of the person so that you can read it with a feeling that they are present in some way.

> **Exceptional Exercise 5.1: Who's on your forgiveness list?**
>
> Where does pessimism, hate or chronic anger exist within you? And whom is it directed towards? Parents, siblings, relatives, friends, your partner (past or present), colleagues, teachers, politicians, war figures, religious figures, sportspeople, and other public figures can all create the toxic, corrosive fluid of pessimism and hate. Start with one, and choose one of the five methods listed in this chapter.
>
> The most important person to forgive in life is yourself. This is the Everest of personal growth for most people. I recommend forgiving yourself once you've worked extensively on forgiving others. Using the analogy from earlier in this chapter, forgiving others will grow your forgiveness muscle enough to then turn attention to yourself.

"Then Peter came to Jesus and asked, 'Lord, how many times shall I forgive my brother or sister who sins against me? Up to seven times?' Jesus answered, 'I tell you, not seven times, but seventy-seven times.'"
– Matthew 18:21-22 NIV

▲ ▲ ▲

Relationship 2: Grandparents

My mum is one of 16 children, the 12th in line. Whilst I regularly thank Mum for giving me life, in many ways I owe my life to a woman I never met: the mother of the first eleven children.

Annie Seymour grew up in the Melbourne suburb of Coburg, next door to my grandfather, Harry Anderson. The two became childhood sweethearts, fell in love, got married and had eleven children together. When Annie gave birth to my auntie Christine, she haemorrhaged and died. By all reports Annie knew she would die in the hours before having Christine.

"Harry told me that just before she died, Annie said to him, 'Who's going to look after my darling children?' And he said, 'Don't worry darling. I'll make sure they're looked after.'" These are the words of my Nana, Norma Anderson (1918–2012). Norma and Harry met in the most peculiar of circumstances. "Our courtship was certainly different to the normal courtship," Nana laughed when I recorded her life memoirs in 2006. "I was leaving St Vincent's Hospital (where she was a nurse) to go for a holiday to see my sister Rose. Sister Mary Fabien (who ran the hospital) rang me and said would I do her a favour – come and meet this gentleman whose wife died and left him with 10 children? [Author note: their first child, Brenda, died at birth].

"The two eldest girls were at boarding school at Genazzano and they wanted new underwear. Mr Anderson didn't want to go buy underwear, as he had not done that before. So I went and met Mr Anderson and we had a cup of tea with Sister Mary Fabien and she said, 'I'll leave you and Mr Anderson to arrange for you to go shopping.' I never did that shopping and I never went to visit my sister Rose. Harry didn't want me to go away."

Four months later my Nana and Pa were married. Nana went on to have five children, the first of them my mum, Clare. Such is the brutal nature of existence, those five children and their respective children and grandchildren all in some way owe their life to Annie's death. My Nana's life purpose would not have materialised had it not been for Annie haemorrhaging.

"When I was 33 I thought I might never get married, which didn't bother me really," Nana recalled. "I didn't even think of having five children." At the time of my Nana and Pa meeting, Nana was being continually persuaded to join the convent, which she declined time and again. When pressed on her reasons for denying her vocation by the nun who questioned her, she affirmed, "Because, Reverend Mother, if I met a man I loved I would get married."

Sometimes you don't think you'll become a parent, let alone a grandparent. But if there's one thing the story of Norma Anderson teaches us, the world works in the most mysterious of ways. If you believe you'll never be a grandparent because you don't have children, think again. You may find yourself in your later years falling in love again or living next to a young family who need the kids looked after on a regular basis. You might volunteer at the local school crossing or in the children's ward at the local hospital. Ignore the role of grandparent at your own peril, because if there's one example that carries through generations more than we'd like to admit, it's the life habits that are formed by our grandparents, passed on to their children and grandchildren.

> **Exceptional Exercise 5.2: Interview your living relatives**
>
> I learnt a great deal about life by interviewing my Nana. If you are fortunate enough to have elderly parents or grandparents, let them share with you their life experiences, their rituals, beliefs, victories and failures. They are living examples of what an exceptional life looks like. Even if they have compromised in some areas of their life, what have you learnt from that? Wisdom abounds in our elders, and it's up to us to glean and incorporate as much of it as we can. A list of questions to ask can be found at **marcuspearce.com.au/yourexceptionallife**

What example are you setting?

Grandparents have the power to set the culture, values and *tone* of the family and future generations. So, regardless of your stage of life, check in and ask yourself the *Eight Exceptional Questions* –

1. Am I doing work that *inspires* me or am I risking *regret* that I didn't do work that I love?

2. Am I moving my body in a way that generates *vitality* or am I risking *cognitive decline* and the chronic diseases that come from a sedentary lifestyle?
3. Am I socially *connected* to a peer group I love or am I in a disempowering peer group or at risk of social isolation and *depression*?
4. Does the food I eat provide me with *energy* or is my diet creating *dis-ease*?
5. Am I a source of love and unity within the family dynamic or am I living with *bitterness*?
6. Am I *enthusiastic*, learning what I love to learn, or am I *bored*?
7. Am I financially *independent*, spending less than I earn and investing the difference, or am I *broke*?
8. Am I *fulfilled*, living with faith in a higher purpose of some kind? Or am I spiritually *broken*?

I ask you this because children notice *everything*. 'Monkey-see monkey-do' does not only apply to manners at the dining table. Your beliefs, spending habits, body language, communication style and all elements of your exceptional life are not just observed by children, but in many cases mimicked and unconsciously accepted as the way to live. If you spend your days watching TV, then it's likely your children will say: "My grandparents sit at home all day watching TV."

What does that do for their view of getting older? It can generate into a global belief that 'older people sit at home watching TV all day'. And when they grow up, what do these children often believe they'll be doing when they are older? "Oh, probably sitting in a home just watching TV all day."

Simply put, if you wouldn't want your grandchildren or future grandchildren to be seeing any areas of your life or behaviour, start changing them immediately. Not moving? Start moving *now*. You will inspire your grandchildren. Are you resistant to forgiveness? Start forgiving *now*; your grandchildren will notice a lighter, happier grandparent. At the grandparent stage of your life, you are not only changing for you, you are changing the legacy you will leave behind. And in many ways, that is more powerful than the impact your decisions have on you alone.

△ △ △

Relationship 3: Siblings

Twins Brielle and Kyrie Jackson were born 12 weeks premature in 1995 at the Massachusetts Memorial Hospital. Brielle weighed just two pounds and was blue-faced from crying so much and was struggling with her heart rate. Gayle Kasparian, the young nurse on duty, asked the twins parents, Heidi and Paul Jackson, if she could do something she had never done before. She asked if she could place the struggling Brielle in Kyrie's incubator. It was a hunch that at the time had no scientific research and had *never* been done before in the US. Twins were routinely kept in single incubators to avoid any risk of infection.

It was then that the unprecedented moment took place. Kyrie, just hours old, wrapped her little arm around her sister. Suddenly, Brielle's crying reduced to sobs and then to nothing; her heart rate improved, as did her colour. Over the following two months, the Jackson twins put on weight, strengthened their little bodies and went home to live a regular life.

Kasparian's courage to follow her intuition, Brielle's dramatic improvement and Kyrie's 'Rescue Hug' as it came to be known, changed the way the entire medical profession treats newborns.

Hugs are necessary even if you're not a hugger

'Double bedding' as it is now known has become common practice for newborn twins. But even more powerful than a change in hospital policy is the power of physical touch. The example of the Jackson twins is that of two siblings, however the 'failure to thrive' phenomenon doesn't just apply to young children; it also applies to adults.

The late Virginia Satir, one of the most respected family therapists ever to live, had a mantra, based on years of research and experience, and it's one that I use over and over again:

"Four hugs a day are necessary for survival, eight are good for maintenance, and twelve for growth."

I love this so much that I apply it at many of my speaking events, and there's one bit of feedback that sticks with me. One attendee wrote down: *I'm not a hugger, in fact I've always avoided it, but after the third hug; I loved it!*

This comment is indicative of where many people find themselves today. If you grew up in a family that doesn't hug, I have no doubt you'll find hugging uncomfortable. Many schools and workplace environments now ban hugging or any form of physical contact, completely oblivious and ignorant of people like Satir's research and the true power of physical touch.

Once in a while we all need a Rescue Hug, and many people simply cannot get it at home – they live alone or in abusive relationships. Wider society is the next best place to get a hug outside of the family home, but sadly many consider it weird, unacceptable or inappropriate to hug a fellow human being.

You may be reading this and have many reasons why you *can't* hug. You may know or live with people with autism, some of whom do not enjoy or respond well to hugging. If you have been raised in a family that doesn't hug or show affection of any kind, I urge you to watch the movie *Temple Grandin* featuring Claire Danes as the autistic Grandin. Introducing small but significant tactile rituals to your relationship can do wonders for your physical and mental health.

Cherish the relationship that may never die

Sibling relationships are the longest-lasting family ties we have. Generous amounts of research suggest that happiness in later life and the quality of relationships with siblings (if you have them) go hand in hand. I have no doubt that this statement will cause resistance for many readers, given that many sibling relationships sour and degrade over time.

Arguments over the family inheritance are perhaps the most common source of degenerative sibling relationships, yet the source of such fractious events often stem back to childhood and early adulthood.

If you felt your sibling(s) received preferential treatment to you, this may play out in destructive ways throughout your adult life.

You may find sibling relationships can break down due to –
- Unresolved pains – from childhood or adulthood and ranging from abuse to deception to perceived favouritism, sweeping things 'under the carpet' only makes matters worse over time.
- Disapproving in-laws – personality clashes with your sibling's partner or relations.
- Lifestyle differences – you drink, they don't; you're vegan, they're not; you live rural, they live urban; you're frugal, they're not; you're a conservationist, they're a chronic consumer.
- Personality clashes – if you have a quiet or peaceful personality and you have a sibling with a loud or powerful personality, clashes and disagreements are often inevitable.
- Different beliefs – about family matters, politics, religion, education, health, etc.
- Money – the inheritance, or even just your financial net worth. You may earn a lot more or less than your sibling, and this can cause tension.

At the same time, there are a number of life events that can strengthen the relationship with your siblings. Just as death can tear families apart, it can also bring families together. Funerals can be very healing events for many people. The breakup of a marriage can also bring people together. I for one can attest to this, as my sisters and I became much closer when our parents split up. Even though I was 10 and my sisters Olivia and Georgia were eight and six, respectively, I can still remember the outpouring of emotion to each other and a shift in the type of love and respect which still exists today.

▲ ▲ ▲

Relationship 4: Intimate Partner

My wife, Sarah, and I could not be any more different. Sarah grew up with two older brothers; I terrorised two younger sisters. Sarah's parents have been married since 1971; my parents divorced in 1991. Sarah grew up in the country whilst I grew up in the suburbs. When we met, Sarah was a chiropractor living an incredibly healthy lifestyle whilst I was a binge-drinking, smoking workaholic journalist. I love a deadline; Sarah hates to rush. I love the noise whilst Sarah craves peace and quiet. I love football and Sarah has no interest in it. I like to stay up late and Sarah loves to go to bed early. We are chalk and cheese in more ways than one, and my bet is that if you have ever fallen in love it has been with someone incredibly *different* to you.

Why is it that after the honeymoon phase of intimate relationships we begin to become annoyed and upset at the very differences that we were first attracted to? The playful fun-loving person you fell in love with is now someone who doesn't take life seriously enough. The caring, detail-orientated angel you were captivated by is now a stuck-up over-analytical devil woman who can find gloom on even the sunniest day.

If intimate relationships teach us anything, it's that all human beings – our partners included – are equal and very different. We are not all the same. No one is worth more than anyone else, yet no one is exactly the same as another. Intimate relationships become difficult when we expect our partner to be more like us; and flourish when we not only accept and appreciate them for who they are, but give up on the expectation that they will change.

Three immovable legs of a relationship

Any seat with three legs relies equally on each leg to keep it upright and perfectly balanced. From time to time chips occur and regular misuse of the seat can create damage. Intimate relationships are no different. There are three legs to an exceptional relationship that each requires equal attention and respect:

1. Your upbringing
2. Your values
3. Your archetypes (including you personality, love language and energy)

Failure to recognise or respect one of these legs may not kill a relationship; but it certainly won't thrive. If you lose respect or awareness of two legs, you may still be able to keep the relationship afloat, but only just. If this is the case, it's more than likely you have emotionally checked out and the relationship exists for conditional reasons only (such as companionship, shelter, finances and children).

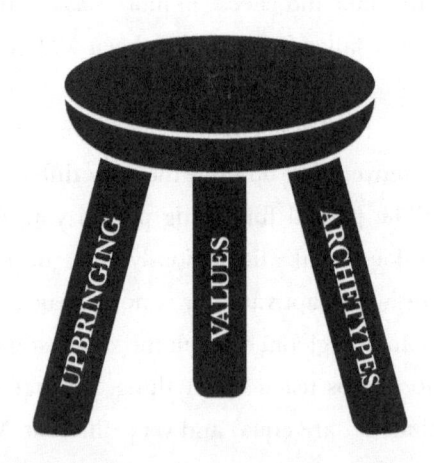

Leg 1: Your Upbringing

The way you were brought up – the town you lived in, the parents you were born to, the siblings you have or did not have, the school you went to, the food you were fed, the house you lived in, the crises you experienced, the friends you made and so on – are 100% beyond your control now. You can't undo your upbringing. Whilst you can alter your perspective about what happened in your childhood, you can never take the events back.

In many intimate relationships you will find that certain parts of your upbringing are quite opposite. Here is a snapshot of Sarah's and my upbringing.

Sarah	Marcus
Public co-ed school	Private boys' school
Country girl	City boy
Quiet house	Loud house
Parents together	Parents separated
Two older brothers	Two younger sisters
Regular camping holidays	Never camped as a family

The differences in our personality which we can largely attribute to our upbringing include –

Sarah	Marcus
Craves peace	Adrenaline junkie
Likes slow	Likes fast
Realist	Idealist
Cautious	Enthusiastic
Sensitive	Not so sensitive
Cries easily	Rarely cries
Early to bed	Late to bed
Quiet (loves silence)	Loud (loves noise)

You may be reading this thinking the above is not relevant to our respective upbringings. I want you to consider though what impact your upbringing, and your genetic imprint, has on who you are. For example, my mum is loud. Nothing Mother Darling does is quiet. My parents split up when I was 10 and my sisters and I lived with my mum. Mum's influence on my life cannot be understated. My upbringing was surrounded by noise! Whether it was loud footsteps or loud jazz music playing, loud conversation or the symphony of pots and pans banging in the kitchen, everything my mum did and still does today is loud. The memories I have of my childhood include singing along to Frank Sinatra's 'Downtown' in the backseat of the car with my sisters; and being five doors down from my home still able to hear Ella Fitzgerald blaring out of Mum's living room.

Can I change this loud part of me? Probably – with *years* of work and therapy! Do I want to? Absolutely not! I love this part of me and it contributes to every part of my life in an empowering way.

Now Sarah on the other hand is not loud. And she has no desire to be loud – the poor soul is married to loud and our kids take after their dad more than their mum in this regard! Sarah's upbringing was far more quiet, and that's the way she likes it. Do I expect Sarah to be more like me? Absolutely not (although I used to – more on that shortly). Does Sarah expect me to be more like her? Absolutely not. And that's why I believe our relationship works.

We do not expect each other to be more like ourselves. We live with, and appreciate the differences we bring to the relationship. We are individual human beings living together. Sarah loves to cry, I rarely cry; Sarah is beautifully sensitive, I am less so; Sarah keeps the kitchen clean as she cooks; I create a mess as I cook. These examples and those listed above are symptoms of our childhood. The challenge you and I have in our adult years is to gratefully accept our childhood and recognise the power and influence it has on us. Unfortunately, most people blame their upbringing for their adult woes, and they bring that baggage into their intimate relationships.

Are you judging or getting frustrated with your partner based on something that has been embedded into them for years whilst living at home? Do they want peace whilst you want ambience? Does your partner want to wait for everyone to be seated before eating whilst you just want to 'eat it whilst it's hot'? These are all likely rituals from your upbringing. Now to be clear, if your partner's upbringing included having the washing done for him or her for two decades and he/she now expects you to do the same, that is not going to fly in the 21st century. This potential grey zone of upbringing is where deep respect and love for each other is essential.

You may remember the story from the introduction that I had a belief that my three-cigarette per day smoking habit was acceptable because it was only three cigarettes per day. Based on my upbringing (my mum also smoked three cigarettes each day), that habit *was* acceptable to me until I met Sarah. Her upbringing and my upbringing were definitely opposed on this one. My love for Sarah and a healthy future together helped me realise that my 'little' habit was over 1000 cigarettes per year and 10,000 per decade, and that rapidly changed my perspective about my upbringing and that 'little' habit.

> **Exceptional Exercise 5.3: Compare your upbringings**
>
> Pull out a piece of paper and write down the elements of your upbringing and that of your partner (if you are currently single use a former partner for the exercise). Consider your school, home environment and location, your parents marital status, employment status, financial habits, dietary habits, siblings, major events or crises, holidays, spiritual or religious beliefs impressed upon you and more.
>
> Have you wondered in depth about what it would have been like for the child version of your partner to grow up the way they did? What did they learn from their upbringing? How has it shaped them? How has it impacted their values, their personality, their beliefs about families and the world at large?

Leg 2: Your Values

Your upbringing will leave an indelible print on what you value most in life and what you value least. Every human being on the planet sees the world differently, and as a result has different values. Our values cause us to dedicate time, money and energy to different tasks, people, goals and decisions. The recipe for what makes up your values has many different ingredients.

For the first 25 years of my life I expected people – everyone – to be more like me and have values similar to my own. I have vivid memories of my frustration as a television and radio journalist, when colleagues wouldn't have the same urgency or adrenaline levels close to deadline. Their calmness made me nervous. I felt as if they didn't care or worse still, were complacent or not aware of the gravity and importance of the situation. With time and further life experience I've come to realise that we don't all need to be ramped up adrenaline junkies!

For years, I unconsciously expected Sarah to have similar values as my own. Those expectations quickly dissolved when I became acutely aware of how different our values were, and how perfect it was that those differences existed.

From the moment our first child, Maya, was born in 2010, I unknowingly expected Sarah to do what I would have done. This related primarily to work. We had our health and wellness centre together, and the business was largely dependent on Sarah to work in order to generate the majority of our income.

When Maya was born we had a locum fill in for three months, thinking that was ample time for Sarah to recover, adjust to life as a mum and return to work.

You can probably see where this is going. Sarah wasn't ready at all to return to work. She was in tears on the way to her first shift back and fought back more tears during each of her appointments. This went on for weeks as the emotional turbulence of starting a family hit a new level. Sarah was juggling motherhood (and the demands of breastfeeding and sleep deprivation) combined with caring for over 150 people each week to help them improve their health. To say that she felt depleted is a massive understatement.

Despite this obvious challenge, I expected Sarah to simply 'switch hats' from mother to chiropractor as she walked through the door (a very masculine trait). This wasn't in Sarah's nature nor in her values. Her highest value was now, unashamedly, family and not work. When Sarah was at work she felt like a bad mother, and when she was at home she still felt like a bad mother because she was so tired. Despite everyone else being in awe of what Sarah was doing, my beautiful wife felt terrible.

She didn't feel at all like the 'superwoman' the community had built her up to be. And here I was, expecting her to live as I would, to just stop 'worrying about it' and switch off. I had completely failed to recognise Sarah's transformational shift in her highest value (from work to family), an event that often takes place after the birth of a child.

> **Exceptional Exercise 5.4:**
> **How To Determine Your Values**
>
> The above example helped me see that my highest value is my work, and Sarah's is the family. Now that may sound mechanical, however once you've worked through this section it will make more sense.
>
> There are many ways to determine your values, and the method I have found most powerful is Dr John Demartini's *Values Determination Process*.
>
> There are 13 questions that uncover your hierarchy of values. From how you spend your time, energy and money, to what you think about and talk about the most, every human being has a different set of answers. Once completed, you will have somewhere between three and nine responses that appear multiple times. In order of what appears most often to least often are your highest values.
>
> You can complete this exercise at **drdemartini.com**
>
> Your list of values doesn't always represent what you necessarily *want* in life. You might want more wealth in your life but your values suggest that you have a higher priority on spending more than saving. You might want more love in your life, yet you find yourself sitting in front of the television more than you do in front of someone else.
>
> Your hierarchy of values demonstrate what you value the *most* and what you value the *least*. Your highest value dominates your mind and your actions. It takes a large chunk of your time and your energy. For me it's my work; for Sarah it's the family.

Your partner has different values to you

I know that each day Sarah is having thoughts that include:

> - *What will I put in the school lunches tomorrow?*
> - *Have I taken the meat out to make dinner tonight?*
> - *How are Maya and Darby getting on at school?*
> - *What activity will I do with Tommy today?*
> - *I really hope Spencer has a big sleep today.*
> - *I need to pull the washing off the line before it rains or else Darby won't have a clean T-shirt for tomorrow.*

In summary, Sarah's thoughts are dominated by the family. I can safely say without shame that none of these thoughts enter my mind each day. Each day my thoughts are dominated by what my highest value is, which is work. I'm thinking about my next speaking engagement or clients, what message I'll share with the crowd, what slides I'll use; what podcast preparation is required, who can I meet with to discuss collaborative opportunities, what book will I read to learn about more exceptional human beings, and so on.

In other words, most of our thoughts relate back to our highest values. And in almost every intimate relationship, the two of you will have a different highest value (for a very good reason). Imagine both of you were dedicated to the family equally. Do you know how often you would butt heads? It would be nigh on impossible to make a decision, as both of you would want *your* way to be *the* way. In our family, household decisions default to Sarah, and business decisions default to me. This setup is in line with our highest values and creates a momentum and harmony that wouldn't exist if we attempted to share the role.

Appreciating the different values

Here is a list of Sarah's and my highest values.

Sarah	Marcus
1. Family	1. Career
2. Nutrition	2. Family
3. Social	3. Wealth
4. Growth	4. Growth
5. Wealth	5. Nutrition
6. Movement	6. Social

What is clear is that Sarah's top value of family and my top value of work is not going to change in the near future. To be clear, Sarah has no intention of working for money in any major capacity in the near future. She loves being a stay-at-home parent and that is the commitment we've made to each other and our family. Despite all the financial gains we would make if Sarah worked, she would be unhappy in the process.

On the flipside, particularly in the early days of starting my business, I was prepared to experience some financial uncertainty and volatility as a result of Sarah being at home. Financial security wasn't worth it if it came at the cost of Sarah's emotional, physical and spiritual health. As you're hopefully learning throughout this book, financial wealth is just one 'asset' of a truly exceptional life. Inspiration, love and health are all far more fulfilling than money in the bank.

So what is great about you and your partner having different values? Using my own relationship as an example, I never have to worry about how our children are being raised. I never worry that they're not getting enough quality time with their parents. I love knowing that Sarah is fulfilling her highest values in an empowered and conscious way. Having gone through the experience of watching my wife work when she'd much prefer to be at home with our children, drives me even more to share my message, grow my business, and fulfil *my* highest values.

I have used the example of my own marriage to demonstrate the importance of appreciating the different values of your intimate partner. My experience is that it's the differences in our relationships that create the quality of our love and connection. If you fall in to the trap of attempting to make your partner 'more like you' or thinking you can change them you're setting yourself up to fail. If your partner was more like you, your attraction would dissipate, your relationship would become unstimulating, and you'd be wanting them to change in order to bring more variety and uncertainty back in to the relationship.

All conflict is a values conflict

Technology is insidious for its easy access. One night whilst dinner was served my beloved Melbourne Football Club was in the midst of a tight battle against Collingwood. If you don't like sport you're probably rolling your eyes at this point! If you are a fan, I'm sure you can empathise. I knew I wouldn't be present at the dining table if I switched off the footy; I'd be thinking about the game and if we were winning. So I did the worst thing possible (for a masculine brain), and attempted to do two things at once: eat with the family *and* keep a sneaky eye on the football. I placed my phone next to the salad bowl, hiding it from everyone's view.

I'm sure you know how this story ends. I was found out within two mouthfuls of dinner by Sarah and my children, and admonished for not being present at the family dinner. They were 100% correct. In that moment I had valued my love of football ahead of quality family time, and it created conflict because it was different to the values of Sarah and the kids. As Sarah said: "If you wanted to watch the football during dinner just say so."

Times of conflict are often the most difficult in a relationship. The first argument is tough, and the 100th is not much easier. No matter how much you love someone, conflict is inevitable because we all live with different values. If you consider your current or former partner, think for a moment what attracted you to them.

Did you fall in love with a man who was successful in his chosen career? Do you now resent how hard he works? Did you fall in love with a beautiful woman? Do you now resent how long it takes her to get ready? Did you love your boyfriend's libido when you first met? Do you now resent that it hasn't left him? Did you fall in love with an extremely socially active woman? Does it now frustrate you that she still has so much time for her friends? Often the values we fall in love with become sources of major resentment if we let them.

This doesn't mean that we need to have similar values – quite the opposite! If that were to happen all attraction would be dissolved. Instead, knowing that any upset or conflict you have with another is due to a conflict of values will help you empathise more with your partner and resolve the conflict before it escalates.

When you recognise that your job in life is *not* to change someone's values to be more like yours, and to instead *appreciate* the differences, you realise that a lot of conflict is avoidable. This in no way means that conflict disappears but if you understand that your anger is nothing more than a values conflict, you won't let those feelings sink in and fester. My experience is that the more we own the belief that we are all different and that we cannot control others, we get better at refusing to let the behaviour of others impact our emotions.

The best type of anger

It's important not to take this so literally that conflict sends you into a mode of indifference and lowered emotional range. Dr Mario Martinez, clinical neuropsychologist and author of the *Mind Body Code*, defines a certain type of anger as a perfectly healthy response in moments of conflict.

"There's certain causes of health and one of them is righteous anger, which means to be angry in a context to protect your innocence or goodwill or that of others," Dr Martinez explained to me on *100 Not Out*. "It's very good to get angry like that but you don't want to make it chronic. You just want to make it contextual. If in a situation you get angry, you let it go after you're done. You don't want to be happy all the time, you want the range of emotions that we've developed as human beings for hundreds of thousands of years."

Righteous anger is not the anger you feel in an effort to be right – it's not about defending yourself on the details of the weather or arguing about if you went on a holiday for six or eight days. Righteous anger is defending your family's name, your community or workplace culture. These are the times to become defensive and angry. And as Martinez explains, it's important to let the anger go when the emotion is over. Becoming chronically angry is no fun to be around.

Where all heartache begins

As Helena, in William Shakespeare's *All's Well That Ends Well* says: "Oft expectation fails, and most oft there where most it promises." To paraphrase, expectation is the root of all your heartache, and most often the expectation is placed on people you love or outcomes that would bring you great benefit. Unmet expectations you have on yourself or others will cause you the most heartache.

You didn't *expect* someone to die, you *expected* your spouse to stay true to the marriage, you *expected* your boss to give you a raise, you *expected* the plane to depart on time, you *expected* your healthy diet to make you bulletproof. Most people live their lives with unrealistic expectations on themselves and others, and as result live in chronic disappointment. When you release or lower your expectations, you reduce your heartache.

I used to expect myself to be happy *all* the time (and therefore I experienced heartache when I didn't feel up and about). As already mentioned, I expected Sarah to be able to go to work and 'switch off' (and then I experienced heartache when she didn't). You may expect your staff or colleagues to behave more like you and care more about their work. You may expect your children to behave like 'good little boys or girls', or your partner to do or say certain things. Most of the time, these expectations are based on what *you* would do in *your* life. We are masters at projecting our own values and expectations on others. And that's when heartache arises.

So what do you do with your expectations? You have two options –
1. ***Communicate your expectations.*** This is particularly important in the workplace and intimate relationships. It's absolutely vital that both parties know exactly what the other wants and expects. It's also a very powerful exercise in understanding your own psyche and belief systems (you'll be amazed how intricate and detailed some of your expectations are).
2. ***Lower or remove your expectations.*** This is a valuable option in relation to people you do *not* know or people you have very little chance of influencing. One example is my Mother Darling. She is loud by nature, extroverted and social. I've never known her to be quiet or reserved. She will never be a wallflower. If you or I *expect* my mother to behave any differently, we will be left disappointed.

The more exceptional option is to simply *love* my mum for who she is, and that is another precious human being. And what's interesting, is when you truly *love* someone for who they are, and you stop trying to change them or expecting them to change, you find yourself enjoying their company even more! In the case of Mother Darling, anyone who knows her will tell you how much fun she is to be around. In a world that is so politically correct, my mum is a breath of fresh air, often saying what everyone may be thinking but too afraid to say. She's great entertainment and a loving, generous soul to boot.

🔺 🔺 🔺

Leg 3: Relationship Archetypes (your personality, love language and energy)

There are hundreds of archetypes and profiles that distinguish all of us as unique individuals. From DiSC® and Myers-Briggs profiles to gender or sexuality, we can be labelled with an identity that some of us love and some of us despise.

In this chapter I'm going to share three archetypes I have found incredibly helpful personally in my marriage and in working professionally with people. They are your personality, your love language, and your energy type.

Do you love structure and find yourself attracted to a laissez-faire unstructured type? Chances are that frustrates you at times! Do you pride yourself on being on time? You may have fallen in love with someone who is late to everything and it doesn't phase them. Do you love your own space, peace and quiet and find yourself in love with an extrovert who craves being around others? These differences in personality are not problems, as many would proclaim; instead they are what make relationships so incredible.

What about the different ways you and your partner feel love? Do you feel loved when your partner says, "I love you" or are you more likely to demand action and say, "Don't tell me you love me, show me"? Perhaps it's neither, and instead you want praise and thanks for all you do, or gifts at the most unexpected times? Or instead of gifts, praise and sweet nothings you want physical intimacy. Foot rubs, massages, hand-holding, cuddles, hair-stroking and lovemaking. Your love language is integral for maintaining and growing an exceptional relationship, and chances are you and your partner have different love languages.

And thirdly, is your core energy masculine or feminine? Do you let go and forget easily or do you hold on and remember everything? Are you deeply compassionate about everything and everyone or are you somewhat detached and unemotional? Chances are your partner is the energy you are not. Masculine energy is attracted to feminine energy, and they aren't always gender-based. You can be male with a core feminine energy, and a female with a core masculine energy. In the LGBTIQA+ community, same-sex relationships still have a feminine-masculine attraction. This energy is the essence of all intimate relationships.

Personalities: When Kim Met Danny

Kim Morrison (b. 1968) is a thought leader on personalities, the author of *The Art of Self Love* and founder of Twenty8 Essentials. In 1990 she fell in love with New Zealand cricketer, Danny Morrison.

"When we first met, I totally loved and appreciated how Danny was so laid back and yet had everything in order, paid bills on time, stacked a dishwasher perfectly and knew exactly where to go whenever we were driving," Kim writes in *Why Can't You Be Normal Like Me*. "He, on the other hand, loved how spontaneous and enthusiastic I was, how I made people laugh and how I always had such a positive cheerful disposition. We fell in love easily and thought it would be unopposed and that way forever. Fast forward a few years when reality actually started to hit us! I began to notice we were annoying one another over silly things. He would nit-pick if I did not know where I parked the car at the shopping precinct or if I seemed to cause chaos in the kitchen with every cupboard and drawer open as I created a cordon bleu meal! He would sit in the car and toot the horn complaining how late we always were if I wasn't ready on time to leave when he was. If I didn't have clear concise instructions he would roll his eyes and just leave me to it. It was frustrating for him – and me.

"I on the other hand thought he stressed way too much, worried about things that he shouldn't and needed to appreciate what I did do well. I told him to lighten up or he would end up with ulcers carrying on the way he did and I personally could not understand how different we were socially where people drained him and did not energise him in the same way they did me! As far as we were both concerned the other was doing these things on purpose just to annoy. It wasn't marriage breaking but perhaps it was heading that way."[12]

The four personalities present themselves

The Morrison love story is no different to billions of others: opposites attracting with a honeymoon period of blissful ignorance to the key differences in personality that would later create monumental clashes and potential angst, resentment and bitterness in the future.

In the 5th century BC, Hippocrates outlined four baseline temperaments – Choleric, Sanguine, Melancholic and Phlegmatic. He observed that each temperament was most affected by one of four bodily fluids: yellow bile (Choleric), blood (Sanguine), black bile (Melancholic) and phlegm

(Phlegmatic). Disease and disability, according to Hippocrates, was as a result of a toxic or deficient amount in each of these four humors.

These four temperaments have been popularised and synthesised many ways over the years. Popular personality profiles Myers-Briggs and DISC all stem from the work of Hippocrates, as do most "four type" frameworks. Morrison focuses largely on the adaptation by Florence Littauer that came to be known as the bestselling *Personality Plus*. She has further adapted the work and wrote her insights in *Why Can't You Be Normal Like Me*.

The four temperaments Morrison refers to are:

> **Powerful Choleric (doer, decisive, loves to lead, strong-willed)**
>
> "Let's do it *my* way" is the catchcry of the *Powerful Choleric*. Independent, decisive, ambitious and goal-oriented, *Powerfuls* are often extroverted natural-born leaders. Historically they were violent, vengeful and short-tempered as they tend to control through anger or the threat of it.

> **Playful Sanguine (talker, creative, enthusiastic, funny)**
>
> "Let's do it the *fun* way" is the catchcry of the *Playful Sanguine*. Highly talkative, active and social, *Playfuls* tend to be extroverted and enjoy being a part of a crowd. Charmers and charismatic, *Playfuls* find it difficult doing nothing and are more likely to take risks.

> **Precise Melancholic (thinker, fact-based, analytical, persistent)**
>
> "Let's do it the *right* way" is the catchcry of the *Precise Melancholic*. The feelers and the deep thinkers, the *Precises* of this world are likely to be introverted and avoid attention of any kind. *Precises* are self-reliant and perfectionists, which can lead to anxiety and OCD-like behaviour.

> **Peaceful Phlegmatic (watcher, diplomatic, balanced, patient)**
> "Let's do it the *easy* way" is the catchcry of the *Peaceful Phlegmatic*. Relaxed, peaceful and easy-going, *Peacefuls* are masters at hiding their emotions and making compromises, often to their own detriment. They are motivated by rest and are sympathetic and accepting.

Personality power

You may already know based on the titles which personality you are dominant in. We have a blend of all four and live in one. In relationships it is highly likely that you will be romantically attracted to personalities *different* to yours. In some cases you will fall in love with someone with a similar personality (it's not wrong, just rare). As a result, it's easy to see why conflict occurs in relationships – we fall in love with people that are so different to us!

When you become aware of your partner's temperament, you then have the power to truly create an exceptional intimate relationship. Applying the knowledge is easier said than done, but the payoff is invaluable.

"Danny and I have learnt how to truly value one another now," Kim concludes. "I can see his need for perfection and being on time is actually a gift to us both. I always pay bills on time now thanks to his attention to detail and he has taught me the art of remembering where I parked the car! What felt like nit-picking I soon discovered was more a need to ensure I didn't hurt myself or make things more difficult. He is just more cautious than me. Danny also knows that cooking for me is an outlet and the kitchen is a place of creation where his cleaning up after me and not saying a word is much more appealing than tutting over my mess. It's fair to say we have learnt to pick our battles and when to let some go."[13]

When you truly love your partner for the temperament and personality they are and have no expectation on them to change, the quality of your relationship skyrockets. Coupled with a deep respect for their upbringing and values, you have the power to create an exceptional intimate relationship.

It's not just your partner's personality that will challenge you. Find out the personalities of your parents, children, siblings, friends, colleagues and people you spend plenty of time with. Navigating your way through these relationships is much easier when you know *how* to relate to the most important people in your life.

Go to **marcuspearce.com.au/yourexceptionallife** to find out which personality you are.

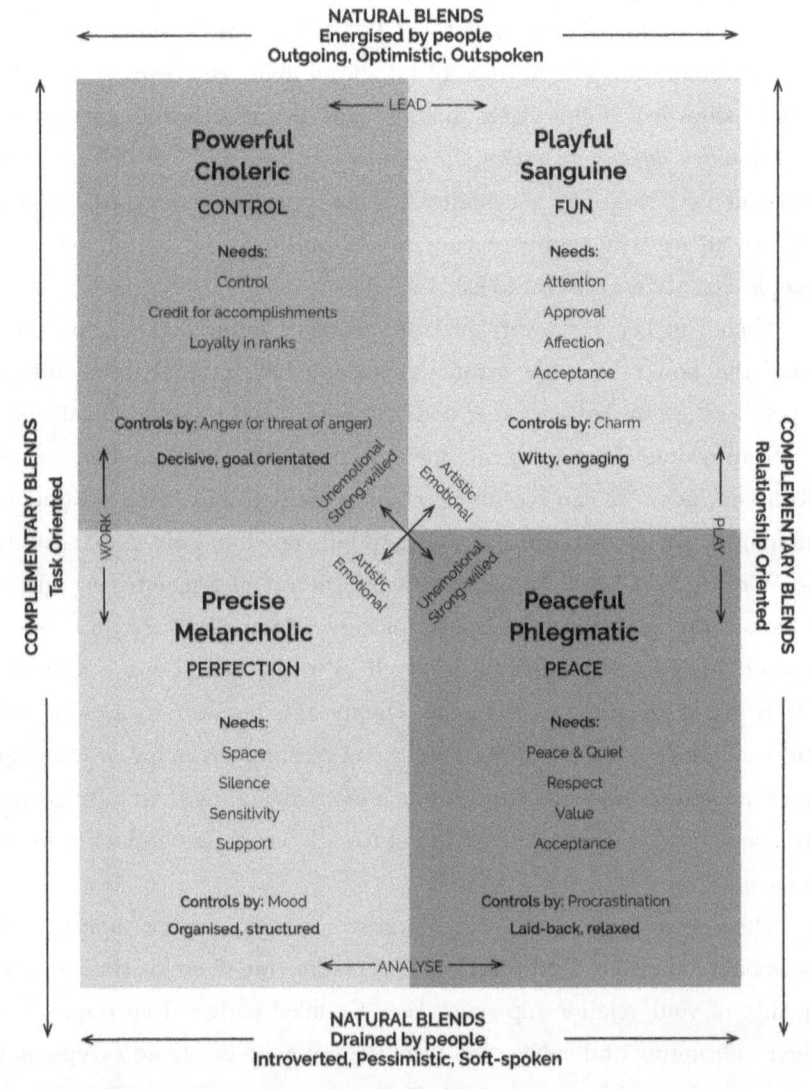

NATURAL BLENDS
Energised by people
Outgoing, Optimistic, Outspoken

← LEAD →

Powerful Choleric
CONTROL

Needs:
Control
Credit for accomplishments
Loyalty in ranks

Controls by: Anger (or threat of anger)
Decisive, goal orientated

Playful Sanguine
FUN

Needs:
Attention
Approval
Affection
Acceptance

Controls by: Charm
Witty, engaging

COMPLEMENTARY BLENDS — Task Oriented ↕ WORK

Unemotional, Strong-willed / Artistic, Emotional

Precise Melancholic
PERFECTION

Needs:
Space
Silence
Sensitivity
Support

Controls by: Mood
Organised, structured

Peaceful Phlegmatic
PEACE

Needs:
Peace & Quiet
Respect
Value
Acceptance

Controls by: Procrastination
Laid-back, relaxed

COMPLEMENTARY BLENDS — Relationship Oriented ↕ PLAY

← ANALYSE →

NATURAL BLENDS
Drained by people
Introverted, Pessimistic, Soft-spoken

Acknowledgement to Florence Littauer, adapted by Kim Morrison

Love Languages

Gary Chapman's seminal book *The 5 Love Languages* applies to any culture, generation, gender or sexual preference. We are all born to love and by virtue of our uniqueness we all feel loved in different ways. And most of the time, the way you feel love is completely different to the way your partner feels love. And by default, what most of us do is give the kind of love to others that *we* love, but our partner doesn't love at all.

According to Chapman, the five ways people feel loved are –

1. *Physical touch* – as little as holding hands all the way up to making love
2. *Words of affirmation* – from 'thank you' to 'I love you'
3. *Quality time* – from chatting over coffee to travelling the world together
4. *Gifts* – from fresh flowers to holidays and houses
5. *Acts of service* – from doing the dishes to making dinner to organising a surprise birthday party.[14]

Do you have a hunch what your Love Language is? If you are in a relationship, do you have an inkling what your partner's is? For clarity, I recommend you and your partner complete the 5 Love Languages quiz at 5lovelanguages.com and share your answers. If you are single, I recommend attempting to fill out the quiz on behalf of your former partner and assess whether a part of the relationship breakdown was due to each partner's love language not being met.

Giving your partner their love language

"If we are to develop an intimate relationship, we need to know each other's desires," says Chapman. "If we wish to love each other, we need to know what the other person wants." Giving your partner their love language is perhaps the great challenge for many in relationship. My love language is *physical touch*, whilst Sarah's is *acts of service*. Can you see how opposite these can be? "Your emotional love language and the language of your spouse may be as different as Chinese from English," according to Chapman. Whilst the idea of constant physical touch is appealing to me, it's not going to fill Sarah's love bucket up. Worse still, it will feel like a burden to her.

Instead, I know that the way Sarah feels love is when I'm *doing* certain things. I make breakfast every morning whilst Sarah goes to the beach or does yoga. On weekends I'll make dinner at least once. I'll do the weekly shop down at the local market so that Sarah isn't darting around town all morning. I'll pick up Maya from ballet and help out with the inevitable children taxi services. If Sarah's feeling off, I'll be with the kids for an hour whilst she goes to the beach for a reset. In other words, whilst Sarah loves a hug and a cuddle, she feels most loved when I am of service to her.

And regardless of what I think of her love language (Sarah doesn't need to *do* anything *for* me in order for me to feel loved), what I know is that giving Sarah *her* love language rather than mine is remarkable for our relationship. And, most importantly, when I give Sarah her love language, she is far more likely to give me *my* love language.

So, do the quiz and find out your own love language and that of your partner's. You can apply *The 5 Love Languages*® principles to almost any relationship. Chapman has also written *The 5 Love Languages*® *of Children* and *The 5 Languages of Appreciation in the Workplace*.

Feminine and masculine energy

Does it drive you wild when your partner comes home from work and has no interest in talking about the day? Or conversely, does your partner want to share every tiny detail of the day whilst you just want to sit and relax? Do you have a partner who tells you to stop worrying whilst you just wish your partner would care *more*? Does your partner forget or let go of things easily whilst you naturally remember the smallest details of random events?

Welcome to the world of masculine and feminine energy, a labyrinth of opposing yet complementary traits that determine attraction and polarity, fuel lust and romance, test unconditional love, and when appreciated and accepted, provide longevity and strength to a relationship.

Whether you've heard it as Yin and Yang, Shakti and Shiva or something else entirely, feminine and masculine energy influences every element of your relationship *and* your life. Being aware of it will save you from avoidable heartache and relationship stress, and at the same time will gift you with an exceptional culture of love.

John Gray's global best-seller *Men Are From Mars, Women Are From Venus* is arguably responsible for putting the differences between men and women squarely on the map. As the years have progressed, however, what's become clear is that it's not as simple to say that men are very different to women. What is more accurate (and relieving for some couples) is that each member of a relationship has a core energy – a typical masculine energy or feminine energy. Yes, most women have a feminine energy at their core and most men a masculine energy, but this isn't always the case. We all have a blend of both, and there is no shame in men having a strong feminine energy and women having a strong masculine energy.

Everyday examples of the masculine-feminine dance

Forgets | Remembers: Masculine energy tends to forget things, whilst feminine energy has an uncanny ability to remember everything! As a masculine male this feminine ability blows my mind, and it often comes up when recalling past events.

Lets go | Hangs on: Masculine energy lives by the mantra 'don't worry about it', which drives the feminine nuts! Conversely, feminine energy is prone to caring 'too much' and not letting go of small and big things. Feminine energy is far more likely to stay too long in toxic relationships.

Path of detachment | Path of compassion: Buddhism outlines two paths to enlightenment: the path of detachment and the path of compassion. Your chosen path in life is designed to cause conflict with your partner as a way to help you create unconditional love and fulfil your potential. If you have a core masculine energy, you likely are more detached, and if you have a core feminine energy you are likely to be on the path of compassion.

Can you see the impending thunderstorm of challenge in intimate relationships? Neither path to enlightenment is better; they are just different. The problem exists when we *expect* others to be on our path and not on theirs. The challenge for the detached is to come closer instead of escaping. Too often the masculine says 'I'll come back when you've calmed down or stopped crying'. Too often the feminine wants the masculine to talk it over, express their feelings and share their vulnerabilities. Loving and respecting our partner for their chosen path is the key.

Makes big things small | Makes small things big: Have you ever been looking at your clothes wondering what you're going to wear today and cracked it because you don't have a clue? Making a small challenge a big drama is feminine energy to a tee (and we love you for it). At the same time, have you had your masculine partner completely shut down or bottle up emotions after a big life event? Anything that 'clears the mind', from watching TV, going fishing, exercising, having a 'quiet' drink with friends (and yes, there's not much conversation) is often the healing path for masculine energy.

As you can see, masculine energy is *very* different to feminine energy. Exceptional relationships depend on our core energies remaining in tact. When relationships lose their polarity or attraction, the breakdown of that relationship begins to occur. Romance descends into partnership, which descends into housemates, or worse into a state of conflict. This slow descent is often insidious, unconscious and almost unintentional. In addition, it's much harder to climb back up the ladder – but it's not impossible and can be done when commitment exists between both partners to reclaim their core energy.

Why relationships neutralise and die

The reason or cause for a loss of polarity or attraction is typically mental and emotional stress. From the daily grind of busy-ness to the crisis and chaos of major life events, we tend to switch energies under these circumstances. If you're a core feminine you become masculine, and if you are masculine you switch to feminine. And if we're not careful, we *remain* in the switched energy for long periods of time without the awareness of what that does to our intimate relationship.

If you know deep in your heart that you are masculine or feminine, you owe it to yourself, your partner, and the people around you to truly own your energy and not to let the stresses of life create an unnatural shift. If you're a feminine female, your best option under stress is to cry (compassionate feminine) rather than to detach yourself (masculine) from the situation. As a masculine energy, I find it far more attractive to see Sarah crying, vulnerable and irrational than stoic, logical and level-headed – all traits which I innately express.

Speaking about masculine and feminine energy with your partner and including it as part of your relationship vocabulary is incredibly beneficial. But more important is your commitment to expressing your core energy and giving permission for your partner to express theirs. When you do this, you unlock the doors to romance, connection and true love that only polar opposites of energy can provide. When you wear a masculine or feminine mask, you not only repel yourself from falling in love, you make it very difficult for your partner to truly express themselves.

Go for progress over perfection

There's a lot to take in here on intimate relationships. Your upbringing, values, personality, love language and energy are all incredibly powerful ingredients in your love life – but resist the temptation to master these all at once. That will only create overwhelm and heartache will ensue as a result of such a high expectation.

Instead, start at the weakest link. Have you failed to acknowledge each other's respective upbringings enough? Compassion and understanding is a wonderful by-product of deep respect for someone's early years. Do you have no idea what each of your values are? Have you been complicit in ignoring your partner's love language and taking the easy road by giving yours only? Is it time to truly understand you and your partner's personality and change the way you communicate and love each other? Or do you need to create a safe space for your core masculine and feminine energy to express itself?

Wherever you begin, start there. No matter how hard it gets, keep working on growing and improving your intimate relationship. When you experience true love for your soul mate, you create for yourself a quality of life that has no substitute.

> *"When there is love, there is no problem."*
> *—Jacqueline Trost*

▲ ▲ ▲

Relationship 5: Children

Artist and author Kahlil Gibran never had children yet wrote perhaps the most powerful message for parents in *The Prophet*.

> Your children are not your children.
> They are the sons and daughters of Life's longing for itself.
> They come through you but not from you,
> And though they are with you yet they belong not to you.
> You may give them your love but not your thoughts,
> For they have their own thoughts.
> You may house their bodies but not their souls,
> For their souls dwell in the house of tomorrow,
> which you cannot visit, not even in your dreams.
> You may strive to be like them,
> but seek not to make them like you.
> For life goes not backward nor tarries with yesterday.
> You are the bows from which your children
> as living arrows are sent forth.
> The archer sees the mark upon the path of the infinite,
> and He bends you with His might
> that His arrows may go swift and far.
> Let your bending in the archer's hand be for gladness;
> For even as He loves the arrow that flies,
> so He loves also the bow that is stable.[15]

I read these pages of *The Prophet* regularly, especially when I'm experiencing challenges with my children. I recommend you ponder the words and consider what each line means for you in terms of your own life and your relationship with your child, or in your relationship with your parents.

You don't belong to your parents, and your children don't belong to you. That is perhaps the most important lesson from Gibran's prose. As parents we can tend to attempt control of our children. As children, we often feel controlled by our parents. If we are to truly reach our full potential and live our exceptional life, we must break free of that control (which is accomplished by living *our* exceptional life to *our* script rather than the script our parents write for us).

As a parent, you must let your child do the same. Your child may love science, whilst you wish they loved art. Your child may want to be a professional singer, which you can't see any future in, wishing instead they became a music teacher or something more 'secure'. Just as Hermann Einstein wanted his son to be an engineer and Florence Nightingale's mother wanted her daughter to be a housewife, attempting to control our children could be holding them back or delaying their true greatness. As a parent your role is to be the archer's bow. Consider what type of bows your parents were. How far and swiftly did they let the arrow be sent forth into the world, and what do their methods teach you about your own beliefs as a parent? How your children choose to lead their adult life and in what profession is not up to you as a parent, no matter how tempting it is to influence and control.

When you bring a heartfelt consciousness to the way you raise your children I have no doubt your relationship with your child – and your own self-esteem – will reach levels you never thought possible.

🔺 🔺 🔺

Family Doesn't Come First for Longevity

Victor Hugo (1802–1885) is renowned as one of the greatest writers of the 19th century. Chances are you've read, watched or attended performances of Hugo's masterpieces such as *Les Misérables* and *The Hunchback of Notre Dame*. At the time of his birth, life expectancy in France was 34 years of age.[16] By the time he died aged 83, life expectancy had crept up to 43.[17] Hugo had five children and buried four of them whilst living to more than double the life expectancy of his generation.

The most tragic child fatality was the death of his daughter Leopoldine in 1843. He discovered the shocking news whilst reading a newspaper during a holiday in the south of France. Leopoldine was just married and taking a boat ride along the River Seine with her new husband Charles Vacquerie, when the boat overturned. Leopoldine was pulled down by the weight of her heavy skirts, and Vacquerie tried in vain to save her life. Leopoldine drowned, and so did her husband. In a heart-wrenching twist, it was discovered the 19-year-old was pregnant. Leopoldine's death broke Hugo's heart. He went into a deep depression from which some biographers assert he never fully recovered.

Countless examples exist from war where entire families have been wiped out bar one or two. The Nazis murdered every member of Eddie Jaku's family except his sister. Grandparents, parents, aunties, uncles, cousins, you name it. Alice Herz-Sommer lived for 72 years without a husband after Leopold died of typhus. If the worst was to happen and your entire family was to be killed, what would you be left with? You'd be left with you, and that's why life purpose comes first in the Exceptional Life Blueprint. The world wouldn't have *Les Misérables* if it weren't for Hugo's heartbreaking life experiences. He began writing the book just two years after Leopoldine's death, and it took 16 years to complete. His anything but perfect family life was a tremendous source of fuel for his literary contribution to the world.

If you find yourself overcommitted to your *family comes first* mentality and with never enough time to look after yourself, you run the risk of sacrificing yourself for the sake of your family. That is the ultimate lose-lose scenario in life, and sadly it happens all too often. For the sake of a great long life, it's important to dedicate your life to what *you* want and not what your family or others expect of you. From premature death, chronic disease and emotional heartache, the consequences can be real and painful.

At the same time, whilst your family won't necessarily make you live longer, it certainly does wonders for your quality of life. Never lose sight of the fact how much richer life can be when love and loved ones are present. Christmas Day becomes a memory-maker rather than avoiding relatives or gearing up for the annual heated family argument. Births, deaths and marriages are far deeper experiences when partners and the wider family get along.

Family comes first in a crisis or special occasion

There are times when family does come first, and it's when special occasions and crises occur. Many hard-working people will put their job to one side to attend a funeral, school concert, a sick family member in hospital, parent-teacher interview, or the birth of their child. At the same time, daily life is littered with examples of these short-term family moments *not* coming first. How many births, weddings, funerals, first days of school, hospital appointments and sports finals have been missed due to work commitments?

No, family doesn't come first in the way people think it does. For many, the notion of *family comes first* is demonstrated by dedicating 80 hours each week to work and provide *for the family*, and the consequence is that they spend very little time with family. The long-term result is that their children get a great education and have a strong foundation for professional life, but perhaps have missed out on emotional connection that may occur in families where work is not such a priority. Immigrant families in particular are littered with inspirational stories of hard-working parents working around the clock to provide an exceptional life for their children in a new country.

So, be clear on what 'family comes first' means to you, and avoid taking it so literally that you need to spend every waking moment with your family. And definitely avoid judging other families for the way they live their 'family comes first' culture. Every family does it differently. To truly own your individual 'family comes first' culture, ensure that your work-family choices are communicated clearly to the family members that are most affected by your decisions.

If you work long hours in your job as a way to provide for your family, it's important to communicate this to your partner and family so that your work is not a source of resentment. If you travel a lot for work commitments, it's important your partner and children know why you travel. For me, my kids know I love my work, and they also know that travelling generates an income for our family to live – to be sheltered, fed, educated and to go on family holidays. They know what it means, and they know that I'm doing it because I love to, as hard as it might be to leave sometimes (particularly when the kids are ill or Sarah is struggling).

A final note on every relationship you have

If you've ever pulled your hair out in frustration at the resistance of others to change, consider for a moment the wise words of Benjamin Franklin –

> *"Consider how hard it is to change yourself and you'll understand what little chance you have in trying to change others."*

Whether we like it or not, taking responsibility for changing other people is not only frustrating, it's futile. Expecting members of your family to change or be more like you not only holds you back, it holds back the other person and your relationship with them.

If you go on a diet, expect to do it alone and not with others. If you want to travel to Paris, prepare yourself that your partner may prefer to go to Bali. If you want to sell your house, don't expect your family and friends to agree with your decision – and resist the urge to convince them that they're wrong and you're right.

Changing yourself often takes time, careful consideration and the facing of fears. Think of any major decision you have made in life and what you went through, and then consider the folly in trying to change others.

When you truly recognise and appreciate Franklin's words you will feel liberated and realise how pointless it is to focus on changing other people. You'll have more energy, more mental and emotional freedom, and more inspiration to dedicate yourself to what *you* really want for your life.

And the best part is that your loved ones will love you for remaining quiet! You won't be a nag or guilty of backstabbing or making passive-aggressive suggestions. You'll be far more fun to be around, non-threatening and a sensational *example* of what it takes to live an exceptional life.

Remember, there is no greater power in life than the example you set. It's the example set by Mandela, Luther King Jr and Mother Teresa that makes us love them so much. It's not because they nagged and judged others. When you simply lead by example by creating and living *your* exceptional life, you create the family relationships you deserve.

GROWTH

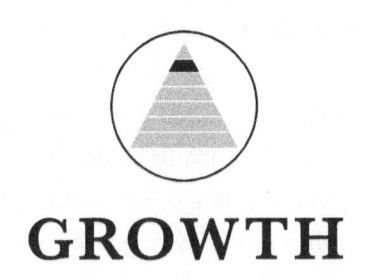

> "Tell me and I forget. Teach me and I'll remember. Involve me, and I'll learn."
> – Benjamin Franklin

Albert Einstein loved to play the violin. Tommy Hafey took his wife to the movies each week and read one book per month. Dexter Kruger turned his hand to writing when his wife died. Sister Madonna Buder first started running at age 48.

Whilst many believe that going to school, getting a job and working for 40 years leaves no time or inclination for growth, *The Exceptionals* see it incredibly differently.

Learning what you love to learn is like a balm for the soul, generating an enthusiasm and *joie de vivre* that no other area of life can deliver. From travelling the world, going to your favourite concert, knitting clothes for your grandchildren or creating a beautiful garden, exceptional growth is more than a hobby; it's a source of inspiration.

On the flipside, next to no growth is the recipe for boredom. The mainstream news, Netflix and social media represent the growth programs for most of us, not only stunting curiosity, but creating a learned helplessness and apathy that most people never wake out of. And with boredom often comes social isolation, the slow emotional death of relationships and a melting pot for poor mental health.

For *The Exceptionals* it's not only what they learn, but how they learn. Most in society are chronic passive learners – watching, reading and listening to information – without any active participation. *The Exceptionals* learn to teach, actively learning their material by speaking, demonstrating and doing the real thing. This active learning embeds the knowledge, generating an enthusiasm and inspiration that passive learning cannot. This chapter is your invitation to unleash your curiosity, quash your boredom and join the few who add this remarkable layer of quality to their exceptional life.

▲ ▲ ▲

Why (and What) Do You Want to Learn?

Englishwoman Sarah 'Paddy' Jones (b. 1934), like lots of young girls, started dancing when she was two. For the next 20 years of her life, Jones took classical dance and a variety of disciplines before giving it up. "I gave it up to get married and had four children," recalled Paddy in 2014 on *Britain's Got Talent*.[1] "I went to live in Spain with my husband (David) and unfortunately after 18 months he died (from leukemia). After David died I kept very busy which is my normal way of life. But I'm not a person for sitting down doing nothing or just watching TV. Dancing had always been my love. So it was what I thought I would go into and try something new."[2]

That 'something new' was a flamenco dance class at the local dance academy owned and operated by Nico Espinosa. From flamenco Jones graduated to salsa dancing and didn't stop there. "Salsa is normally Latin-American dance with your feet firmly on the floor," Jones explains. "But *Salsa Acrobatica* is when the male partner lifts you, throws you, puts you through his legs, over his shoulder and does all sorts of positions and the girl is just there to go into beautiful positions all the time. It's not for the faint hearted!"[3]

Paddy and Nico became dance partners and in 2009 showed their moves on the Spanish talent show *Tú sí que vales*, claiming top prize. Five years later, at 79 years of age, Paddy was again joined by Nico on *Britain's Got Talent*. Before they started dancing, judge David Walliams sniggered: "This reminds me of a *Little Britain* sketch."

Taking my television producer hat off and putting scripted production values to one side, Walliams's tone was ageist and somewhat mocking of a 79-year-old woman dancing with a man half her age on national television. Judge Simon Cowell buzzed the pair out early on in their performance just moments before the *acrobatica* part of the salsa came alive. To rapturous applause, gasps and roof-raising pandemonium, Paddy and Nico gave the performance of a lifetime to simultaneously silence and inspire the critics and provide the perfect example of what exceptional growth looks like – at any age. Judge Amanda Holden gave Paddy and Nico her 'golden buzzer' – a straight passage through to the final, where they finished ninth.

The seeds of exceptional growth were often planted in childhood

Jones, who has officially claimed the Guinness World Record as the world's oldest acrobatic salsa dancer, has an enthusiasm and reason for dancing that stretches beyond curiosity of the unknown. Instead, her exceptional growth is a matter of unfinished business from her childhood and a just reward for her sacrifices.

"When I started to do this I spoke with the family and I said, 'What do you think?' And they said, 'You gave everything up to have us and look after Dad, and he would be proud.'"[4]

Whilst society may call Jones's love affair with dancing a hobby – something we do with our spare time (whatever spare time is) – exceptional growth is defined by an enthusiasm that a small hobby simply cannot provide. Exceptional growth lights a fire in your heart and brain and has a magnetism that you can't help being attracted to.

To find this magnetism and enthusiasm is not as difficult as it sounds. What it takes is some time and reflection and a tiny dose of courage to do something you haven't done in many years (albeit that you loved to do). The first place to go looking is your childhood, as Paddy Jones did. Her story is like millions of others: the young adult who felt the need to suppress childhood passions due to playing 'grown ups' (work or family commitments), only to then retire and/or have an empty nest and more time to fill. Sadly, most people don't put the effort in to seeing it this way, instead filling their time with eight hours of TV each day and pottering around doing very little.

Personally, I feel like I gave up French and piano too young in my life. To this day I still have an enthusiasm and curiosity for them that I am yet to satisfy. Travelling to France only whets my appetite to master the language, whilst helping my children play the piano keeps me wanting to improve at it.

Is it time to resume the stamp collection you stopped in secondary school when homework intensified? Is it time to become a true greenthumb, join the local choir or resume violin lessons which ended 40 years ago? Exceptional growth isn't just about passing the time, its intention is to light you up in a way no other area of life can.

*"No matter what your age or your life path…
it is not too late or too egotistical or too selfish
or too silly to work on your own creativity."*
– Julia Cameron

What brings you pleasure can reduce or eliminate your pain

Professor Marc Cohen (b. 1964) is a medical doctor with degrees in physiology and psychological medicine. A board member of the Global Wellness Summit, Cohen shared on *100 Not Out* that his clinical experience taught him the power of exceptional growth on healing. "One of the most key questions I used to ask my patients was 'what was the most fun you've had in the past week, month or year?' Or 'what activities totally absorb you in the activity?' As health practitioners," Cohen continued, "we are told to ask all about pain – the site, the severity, whether it radiates, what are the onset and offset relieving factors and all these other things – but it's very rare that we ask about pleasure, and it's just as important.

"When you ask people what turns them on – where do they get their pleasure in life and what makes them tick – you literally see them change in front of you. When they start talking about the things that matter to them, their eyes start to sparkle, their voice becomes more enlivened, their posture changes. So even in the short space of a consultation you know that you've hit something that matters to them because they actually enliven – they become more alive in front of your eyes.

"Very often you could track the worsening of their disease or condition to when they stopped doing the things they loved. People think 'I have to give up time for my kids or my job' or 'my illness is preventing me from doing the thing I love'. I used to find out what they loved to do and write a prescription for doing that. So I used to write prescriptions for ballroom dancing and making model aeroplanes, or whatever it was for that person. I'd put it on a script pad and give it to that person and ask them to put it on the fridge and say, 'You need to do this three or four times per week'. People would think I was crazy initially, but then I'd explain to them that this is really important for your health and then they were actually quite grateful.

"By giving them permission to do the things that enlivened them, that really helped manage their condition. You'd also do other things (medically) that would help manage their condition as well, but getting people to engage more in life (is important). I'm a big fan of Joseph Campbell and I would often say to my patients, 'follow your bliss'. You have this internal compass that tells you what the right thing to do is at any moment. So if you give permission to actually enable people to do that, you enliven them. In enlivening them you're going to give them the best chance at living a long life."

▲ ▲ ▲

How to Learn

There are many ways to learn these days. We can read books, listen to podcasts and watch movies. We can attend lectures, workshops, seminars and retreats, or immerse ourselves in apprenticeships and trainings. And that's just the beginning. What differentiates all learning is whether it's active or passive.

Given how much choice we have today, we easily forget that passive forms of learning such as reading, listening and watching is not where the bulk of learning takes place. What we watch, listen to or read may plant the seed of a great idea inside of us – which is what I love about them – but they don't create or embed the skill. Instead, chronic passive learning is the playground of the 'know-it-alls'.

"I don't believe knowledge is power at all," according to learning expert Jim Kwik, author of *Limitless*.[5] "It has the potential to be power but all the podcasts, online programs, coaching, seminars – none of it works unless we work it."[6]

In order to truly learn anything, we must cross the big scary bridge from passive learning to active learning. Active learning requires you to get off the couch or out of the house or up from the desk. Active learning includes speaking about the topic, giving a presentation and doing the real thing (as obvious as that sounds). Retention of information is far greater when you combine passive learning with active learning. As an example, researching for this book has been a passive form of learning, whilst writing the book and speaking about it has been an active form of learning.

If you listen to a podcast in French (passive) and then speak some French shortly after (active) you will learn French much more easily and quickly. If you read a book that opens your mind (passive), the exceptional step is to *talk* about what you learned and apply the learnings. Book clubs are wonderful for this very purpose and are a great example of exceptional growth combining with exceptional socialising.

The secret to exceptional growth is to be an active learner. Jan Smith didn't just read about Everest, she went there and scaled the summit at 68 years young. Supercentenarian Dexter Kruger didn't just *think* about writing books, he jumped the bridge from passive to active and started writing himself. Reading the books and brochures about your favourite travel destinations won't get you there – they'll plant the seed and water it for a while – but nothing completes the learning experience like doing the real thing and getting on that plane.

If you aren't growing, you're dying

Socrates proclaimed: "The only true wisdom is to know that you know nothing." It sounds like a brutal insult to your intelligence when taken literally, but said another way by McDonald's founder Ray Kroc: "As long as you're green, you're growing. As soon as you're ripe, you start to rot." When you lose the attitude of the student and behave like the master, you begin the rotting process. Every master you love and respect is likely to have been a lifelong learner and student of their craft.

The alternative is to be the 'know-it-all'; the person who *knows everything* when really they are shut off from any form of active learning apart from speaking. The mindset of knowing and completion is akin to rotting. When you feel like you know enough, you subconsciously shut yourself out from growth. The exceptional artist wants to be a better painter. The exceptional reader wants to read more books. The exceptional teacher wants to educate in more masterful ways. The exceptional gardener wants to learn new techniques or plant something new. This perpetual desire to grow in the areas of our curiosity lives in all of us, but only *The Exceptionals* let it express itself.

I remember attending an event where the presenter said, "If you think you've got your life sorted, it's time to dig deeper." Living your exceptional life is a lot like that. If you think you've mastered all eight areas of your life, it's time to dig deep enough to become vulnerable again and identify where curiosity abounds. Moments of contentment are wonderful and to be enjoyed, but too much of it becomes boring and stifling. Gandhi proclaimed that a "healthy discontent is the prelude to progress", which is a far wiser attitude to have in growth and in life.

The Exceptionals are never quite content with their output. Dexter Kruger wants to write until the day he dies; Jan Smith wants to scale the seven highest mountains in the seven continents on the planet. Compare this with the alternative of passing time in front of the TV or getting to the end of your social media feed. There are empowering ways to grow and disempowering ways to grow; the choice is yours.

Age is no excuse to stop learning

Dexter Kruger writes his books in long hand first and because he's blind he can't read his writing, so the writing is almost completely illegible. "I just have a look at the scrawl," explained Kruger's writing aid and informal editor Janet Rowlings.

"If I can make out a word here or a word there, that just prompts him to pick up the story. So that's quite amazing. Once he gets on a roll he just goes for it and I'm going 'hang on, hang on' while I try to keep up with him. I've often said to him just to dictate but he can't work like that."

With 12 books to his name and 111 candles on the cake at the time of print, the retired farmer from Roma in Queensland is proof you are never too old to start something new. "I started writing a couple of years after my wife passed away. With no one to talk to in the evening I began writing some stories and now I have an album with eleven books in it and it's called *Dexter Kruger's Stories*," he says.

Take a leaf out of Dexter's books and refuse to let your age define your next area of exceptional growth. When major chapters in our lives come to an end – our work ends, the children leave home, and relationships end – great opportunity exists. These times can be the beginning of something magnificent. You could do as Ruth Frith did and start athletics in your seventies, or as Charles Eugster did and hit the gym in your eighties. "Go make yourself necessary," is what Dr Walter Bortz was told by his father growing up. Just as Bortz believes with exercise we must also believe for growth: "It is never too late to start; and always too early to stop."

> *"As soon as you say you can't do something,*
> *you begin to grow old."*
> *– Wang Deshun*

> **Exceptional Exercise 6.1: What do you want to learn?**
>
> Here's your opportunity to create a plan for your own exceptional growth. What exceptional growth do you want to experience? What will bring out your enthusiasm and curiosity like nothing else? Is it travelling, learning a language or an instrument, or building something?
>
> Remember, passive learning is *necessary* to the process. Learning the fundamentals of any topic often begins in a passive form. If you want to travel to France, you'll want to passively learn about the language basics, currency, culture, time zones, modes of transport, accommodation and food. You'll prepare yourself for all of these things. Then, on an *active* level, you start to learn the basic words and phrases.
>
> The best part of course, is 'doing the real thing', landing in Paris and if you're lucky, heading out to the villages and experiencing *true* France (clearly I'm biased).

Immerse yourself in all forms of learning

When you consider how many ways there are to passively and actively learn, you'll find a vast array of experiences to deepen your learning about anything. Take music for example. There's listening to your favourite song, reading the lyrics and mastering them, singing the song, watching the song's film clip, dancing to the song and then dancing to the song with others. And if you're lucky, there's singing and dancing to the song with others at the live concert of your favourite performer. They are all incredibly different learning modes and when you combine them all together you truly get an exceptional growth experience.

Combining growth with movement and socialising

For many *Exceptionals* their growth is an opportunity to move and socialise at the same time. In many longevity cultures, gardening is a hobby that is not only a passion but is also sensational for physical health and vitality. Bending, stretching, lifting, balancing, getting in awkward positions, using the hands, and so on are all vital ingredients for the body. In addition, when it's done with family and friends, and also combined with a good meal together, you can see how one area of your exceptional life can easily incorporate many others. The ultimate gardening experience incorporates exceptional movement, social, nutrition, family, growth and arguably wealth (saving money), spirit (connection to nature) and you could easily declare it beneficial to an exceptional life purpose.

A word on technology

No one can argue that technology has radically improved our ability to grow and be educated in any subject. COVID-19 brought to light not only how much we rely on technology, but gave humanity the opportunity to socially connect through technology, learn something during times of isolation, and even launch new businesses, or to reframe existing ones.

When pandemics aren't taking over the planet though, the balance of the role technology plays is much finer. Importantly, *The Exceptionals* embrace it. "Mental stimulation is important. I have a computer and a smartphone," Heather Lee, the world's fastest female walker over 90, shared with me on *100 Not Out*. "I've really kept up with the times, which I think is really important. I've seen quite a few things, having survived the war in England. Adapting to the times is challenging but I love a challenge. I can send photos but I'm not into the apps. I only use it for what I need it for."

If you're 'up with the times' like Lee, the trap to watch out for is the passive learning vortex that technology keeps many people in. Passive learning is so compelling and visually attractive that it makes active learning seem unnecessary. Well-produced learning programs, incredible documentaries, entertaining podcasts and beautiful infographics all have their place, but nothing will teach you like doing the real thing.

When you know what you're curious about and from where your enthusiasm springs, you'll feel the uncertainty and fear that crossing the bridge from passive to active learning is supposed to provide. This is a test to your spirit and will to experience the exceptional growth you deserve. Use the Susan Jeffers mantra: "Feel the fear and do it anyway" and exceptional growth is yours for life.

> *"The older I get, the less I know. It's wonderful –*
> *it makes the world so spacious."*
> *– Swami Chetanananda*

▲ ▲ ▲

The News

Nothing represents mediocre growth more than our toxic appetite for news. Not only is our news consumption the epitome of passive learning (watching, reading and listening), we defend our news habits like children fighting over lollies in a piñata. Being informed may seem essential to most of us, but what if the issues we're informed about are contributing to our struggles in other areas of life? Many of us are more informed about celebrity relationships than our own marriages; we know more about our favourite sporting teams than the sports our children play or the subjects they're studying at school.

10,000 stories per year

It's estimated that we consume approximately 10,000 news stories per year, or 27 per day.[7] If you find this number to be high, consider how many stories you consume through television, social media, radio and print media (both online and offline). With the rise of social media as a news source, that number may in fact be closer to 20,000 per year and more than 50 per day. Consider for a moment how many of those stories have helped you live a more exceptional life, and my tip is the answer would be very few, if any.

News stresses us out

"If it bleeds, it leads" is the catchcry of many a newsroom. In other words, the worst news is the highest priority and the cat stuck up a tree goes last. Unnerving and 'shocking' stories spur the release of cortisol in the body. Cortisol is a hormone which can be very good for you at certain times – it's responsible for waking you up each day – but when released constantly, cortisol has a toxic effect. In short, cortisol is the primary stress hormone in the body. And when we stress, our digestion and immune systems are impaired, whilst mentally and emotionally we are more fearful, anxious, depressed, aggressive and desensitised. If you already have enough stress in your life, going on a news diet is a quick and easy way to lower your cortisol levels and claim back some calm.

> *"There's mass media, then there's more masterful media.*
> *By the time the truth puts on its shoes the*
> *illusions spread across the world."*
> *– Dr John Demartini*

Stop eating the news for breakfast

Even if you think news doesn't affect you, choosing to consume the news as soon as you wake up is a mediocre start to the day. I'm sad for people who have been murdered and their affected families; I'm sad for people who have died in car accidents and I'm sad for the millions of people displaced through the atrocities of war and terrorism. I'm sure you are too. I don't though, need to bombard myself with this knowledge just moments after waking up. Unless you're a leading politician or superintendent of police, neither do you.

Consider for a moment that the news triggers the limbic system, the part of the brain responsible for functions including emotion, behaviour, motivation and long-term memory. Is it really worth feeding your emotional regulator a steady diet of bad news for breakfast?

What if you started the day by writing the news of *Your Exceptional Life*? "A middle-aged woman in her 40s was seen waking up at six o'clock this morning to go for a walk with her friend. After a brisk 30-minute session, the two were then seen returning to their respective homes and preparing the family for the day ahead." Nothing newsworthy there, except that the two women have ticked off exceptional movement and social life and are about to begin family, nutrition and life purpose.

One of the quickest and easiest ways to dampen your soul and lose your inspiration for daily life is to be a regular consumer of the mainstream media. To fill your mind with the novelty of murder, tragedy, death, war and hate is but one side of the story of life. If this is pushing your buttons, please know that I'm not having a go at you for watching the news. I just want you to write the script of *Your Exceptional Life*, and it's difficult to do that when the mainstream media is constantly by your side to help you write it.

> *"Create before you consume."*
> *– Marie Forleo*

Is there any news that does benefit?

The only news that benefits or has zero (or minimal) toxic effect is the news that doesn't negatively impact your emotions. For me, sports results and match analysis fit in to this category. For you, it might be business or industry news. Other interests including travel, the arts and entertaininment, food and gardening are unlikely to trigger negative emotions, unless you use them as a source of comparison. If that is the case I would recommend you reduce or eliminate their consumption.

It's the 'top' of the news that you are wise to be wary of. The child murdered by her parents; the threat of war, the rise in violence, racial tension, and so on. Most of the time, the top of the news is completely outside of your control. These stories will not help you live your exceptional life.

If you love where you live and are inspired to help your community, being aware of local news can be incredibly valuable. But again, be wary of local newspapers. Many of them are owned by multinational media companies and still have a culture of sensationalism, even of local news.

Choose your own media

So what's the solution to all this naysaying of the news? The answer is simple, easy and fulfilling: choose your own news. It is easier today than ever before to control your own media consumption. You can listen to, watch and read essentially *anything* you want at *any* time.

Video streaming services such as YouTube and Netflix have become TV on demand. Podcasts now allow you to pause, fast-forward, rewind and even speed up or slow down any piece of content. Most radio programs will now publish their entire shows as a podcast. The internet now allows you to learn whatever you want whenever you want, rather than being limited to one or two newspapers in your city and a local library. Add to this the millions of online courses available (many of them provided free by leading universities around the world), and we truly have created a 'knowledge on demand' global society of information.

But please never forget the power of a good book. Books, outside the real-life guidance of an elder, are arguably the greatest teachers we have on the planet. "Books are the quietest and most constant of friends," said Charles W. Eliot, former Harvard University president. "They are the most accessible and wisest of counsellors, and the most patient of teachers."

"If you don't like to read, you haven't found the right book."
– J.K Rowling

Never forget the most important news

Remember that your own news and that of your family and friends is more important than the news of the country or the world. Longevity cultures spend their evenings immersed in long dinners, socialising with friends and family, discussing the news of their local community and each other (and of course at times the news of the world). You can do this too – virtually or in person. It takes nothing more than a cup of tea or glass of wine (the drink really doesn't matter), and an authentic priority of the other person over the television or social media. The conversation could be deep and meaningful or completely trivial. Again, it doesn't matter. What matters is that you are more informed about the people you care most deeply about than the people you'll never lay eyes on.

"A room without books is like a body without a soul."
– Cicero

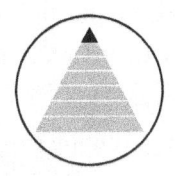

WEALTH

"A feast is made for laughter, and wine maketh merry: but money answereth all things."
– Ecclesiastes 10:19 KJV

The most harrowing picture I have of old age is not of an impoverished elder in a developing country. It's of an 80-year-old with dementia, sitting up in bed in a nursing home. She is sitting in her own urine because the facility she lives in is underfunded and simply doesn't have the staff resources to supply even the most basic of support. And the brutal reason why this person is spending their final years in that home is money, and the lack of it.

This scenario could be often prevented through a combination of elements – exceptional movement, social and family relationships to name but three – which I've covered previously. This is a chapter on wealth, and sadly most of our elders have not managed their money well enough in their life.[1] As a result, up to 85% of their pension goes to aged care accommodation, they sit in a room with few to no visitors and suffer a sadly undignified final end to life.[2]

If you only achieve one thing from this chapter my wish would be that you gain the financial independence to enjoy a dignified end to your life, surrounded by family and friends in an environment that is clean and comfortable and on your terms. In order for this to happen, your relationship with money may need to change.

Just as key figures in your upbringing can heavily influence your career and relationships, so too can they take hold of your wealth philosophy. Can money make you happy? Are rich people bad people? Is wealth a dirty word? Your answers quite possibly were given to you whilst growing up and will appear today in your net worth. Do you spend less than you earn? Do you have seemingly insurmountable debts? Do you know how much it costs to run your life? Do you have a long-term vision for your financial wealth? Do you feel guilty about money? Your answers to these questions are the key to unlocking your exceptional wealth.

For many, discussing money and wealth is a taboo topic. This chapter is dedicated to breaking the shackles and having a deep and meaningful conversation about your exceptional life and the role wealth plays in it. Money is nothing if not a great amplifier of who you are and what your life is about. Forget about the decisions you've made in the past. Start with a blank canvas, and fiercely recognise that the decisions you make from this day forward will impact your financial destiny and your exceptional life more than you will ever know.

▲ ▲ ▲

The True Meaning of Wealth

Imagine this: four coffee-loving people are given a $10 Starbucks gift card. Amidst their excitement at a free Pumpkin Spice Latté or Green Tea Crème Frappuccino, they are each told there's a catch: each person must use their gift card differently.

Person One is instructed to use the gift card personally.

Person Two is instructed to take someone else out for coffee.

Person Three is instructed to gift the $10 voucher to someone, but they are not to go to Starbucks with the recipient.

Person Four is instructed to take someone else out for coffee, but use the voucher on themselves only and not the guest.

Which person do you think was the most fulfilled? Do we get our pleasure from buying things for ourselves, sharing our things with others, giving things away passively or showing off our good fortune? This exact experiment was conducted by Lara Aknin of Simon Fraser University and featured in Elizabeth Dunn and Michael Norton's book *Happy Money: The Science Of Smarter Spending*.[3] This part-social, part-financial experiment found that person two – who took someone else out for coffee – enjoyed the most fulfilment, demonstrating how giving our money away can in fact be a great source of happiness.

Dunn and Norton add that there are three major ways that money can bring happiness:

1. **Investing in others** – as previously shared, giving our money away makes us happy!
2. **Investing in experiences** – travelling, learning new skills or doing some form of personal growth are all rewarding and fulfilling.
3. **Buying time for yourself** – here's where outsourcing your most dreaded tasks brings you fulfilment. Cleaning, gardening and accounting are just three examples. The fulfilment lies in not just outsourcing, but in using that time on yourself. You might get a massage, catch up with friends, go to the movies, or go walk your favourite trail.[4]

Whilst I typically get a room full of people split down the middle when asked if money can make you happy, when I outline these three examples of what money can buy, no one disagrees.

Why the poorest people are often the happiest

At the same time, the world's poorest aren't investing their money in experiences or delegating their least favourite tasks to others. So what's their secret and how do we replicate it? Why is it that many people with little material or financial wealth are happy?

The answer lies in the clear distinction and separation of your self worth from your net worth. The happiest people don't *need* money to be happy or fulfilled; financial and material wealth doesn't define them. They are already multi-billionaires in the first six areas of their Exceptional Life Blueprint.

Let's take Joanna, the delightful Ikarian elder featured in the movement section, for example. Joanna fills her days with activities that provide her with purpose – checking in on neighbours and family, picking grapes from the vine, making cheese, cooking and so on. She tends the garden, sweeps the patio and walks down dozens of jagged steps to run errands in the village (movement), where she spends time with family and friends (social). She eats the traditional food and has ceremony around meal times (nutrition), remains connected to her husband, Giannis, and extended family, and remains curious and open to learning (growth). Financial wealth, whilst it could possibly make life easier for Joanna, does not guarantee her any more fulfilment than she already has.

For traditional communities in developing nations, too much material wealth is quite deleterious. A television is introduced to the village and the community moves less. Children and adults alike become less social, become more disconnected from each other and embrace less of their environment and culture. It was only the material wealth (or the donation of material wealth) that caused this slippery slope. The same could be said for smartphones and even automobiles in some countries or cultures where that type of travel is not common.

In Ikaria, there is very little cultural focus on material wealth. You won't find a brand-new Mercedes or BMW anywhere on the island of 7,500 people. Not one. On my first trip to Ikaria I was told of an American who had decided to retire on the island and buy herself a new BMW as a gift. Within four weeks of acquiring the car she sold it back to the Athens car dealer, fully realising that not only was she the only one on the island with a brand new BMW, the car didn't give her anywhere near the fulfilment that she thought it would.

You're wealthier than you think you are

If you are reading this book you are incredibly wealthy. Just having the means to buy it puts you in the top 4% of the global rich list, and if you can also speak, read and write, you truly are beyond gifted to live the life you lead. You are not one of the more than three billion people living on less than US$5.50 per day.[5] Take a moment to visualise what three billion people really looks like – to give you an idea it's 30,000 Melbourne Cricket Grounds filled to capacity. Then consider what US$5.50 per day really looks like and how fortunate you are.

You are likely not one of the 500 million Indians who live without electricity and fresh water. You are likely not in the middle of a genocide in your country. It is highly likely that the biggest financial problems you face each year are how to finance a family holiday or pay the mortgage, improve from five to six figures, or six to seven and beyond. You probably have what we like to call 'first world problems'.

Almost half the planet lives off three figures per year. Never, ever forget the gift of a meal, the gift of a good night's sleep, and the gift of a smile from a loved one. It is a privilege to be alive in the world we live in. Not only do we have the opportunity to live our exceptional life, we have, as Seth Godin emphasises in his book *Tribes*, an *obligation* to do so, given the opportunities we have. You are obliged to use your position as one of the fortunate ones to help humanity live their exceptional life. That can be in the way you raise your own children, help your colleagues, engage with your community or give to charity. This is not a purely financial obligation; it's in your intent and awareness that true wealth really shines. And sadly that's where so many people get it wrong.

Do What You Love to Earn What You Love

"Follow your passion," says Oprah Winfrey and countless other *Exceptionals*. "Do what you love, and the money will follow. Most people don't believe it, but it's true." The reason why most people don't believe it is because they're expecting the money to follow immediately or soon after. For *The Exceptionals*, they're prepared to follow their passion for years – even decades – before seeing the money follow.

Reality television shows are littered with examples of people who have 'followed their passions' for years without any financial gain. In 2009, Scottish woman Susan Boyle begrudgingly entered *Britain's Got Talent* (BGT) at the behest of her vocal coach. She'd previously withdrawn from auditioning on *X Factor*, believing she was not pretty enough, and almost withdrew from BGT, believing she was too old. Her dream of being a professional singer had been with her since she was five years of age.

Just like the aforementioned Paddy Jones, Boyle was given a cynical, mocking welcome by the judges and crowd at her audition. Not only did Boyle wow the judges and a nation with her performance of *I Dreamed A Dream* from *Les Misérables*, she went on to come second on BGT and launch her professional career at the age of 47. That's right; 42 years – six cycles of seven – after first dreaming of being paid to sing, Susan Boyle realised her dream. Boyle has gone on to sell over 20 million albums and has a net worth of over 22 million pounds. Her commitment to do what she loves, despite her fears, has paid off handsomely.

The most fulfilling way to earn money is by doing what you love to do. When you spend your working hours doing activities that bring you joy, being paid for it seems like a bonus rather than an entitlement or reward for effort. For me, the penny didn't drop until 2011 when Dr John Demartini suggested to me that if I loved talking so much "maybe you could make a career out of it". Today, the most profitable arm of my business is speaking. Interestingly, I could do it all day and be paid nothing for it. I simply love talking about living an exceptional life. Creating exceptional wealth by doing what you love is not a coincidence; it's simply an effect of persistence combined with the dedication of time.

What would you do with your life if you didn't have to 'pay the bills'? *That* is the very activity your working hours are ideally consumed with. Whilst you may resist and say, "but Marcus I *do* have to pay the bills," simply beginning with five, 10 or 30 minutes a day of this activity will bring you great joy and fulfilment and plant the seeds for future financial wealth. Whether you call it a side hustle, second job or passion project doesn't matter. What matters is the feeling you get from spending time doing more of what you love. When you do that, you generate the ideas, tenacity and commitment to earn what you love by doing what you love.

Only one word of caution applies here. If you believe your passion is more of a hobby, I recommend keeping your hobby just that. If you risk losing love for something that brings you joy, then that is not the career for you. I love playing the piano, but there is no way I want to be a professional pianist. If, however, you love the idea of being paid to sing, make soap, complete tax returns for other people, clean houses, make clothes or whatever your passion is, then know that your greatest potential for exceptional financial wealth lies in doing what you bounce out of bed for each day.

But isn't too much money a bad thing?

One of the reasons people stop themselves from creating greater wealth is their belief that money is bad; or at least too much money is bad (however you define too much).

One of the more widely known rags to riches story of wealth is Oprah Winfrey. With a net worth of almost US $3 billion, Winfrey is certain money hasn't changed her as a person. "I'm not acting like 'oh gee money isn't important' and all that, because it does add a certain level of comfort to you," she reflected in 2017. "But this is the real truth, wherever you are in your life, if you win the lottery you will still be the same person, and that money and those things you will now be able to buy are just a magnifying glass on who you already are."[6]

I think most of us would agree that Oprah Winfrey is a good person, and money gives Oprah more to be *good* with. The Oprah Winfrey Leadership Academy for Girls in Johannesburg is just one example of Oprah's wealth being used for good. With over 300 students enrolled, the OWLAG has given many young women the "potential to be an Oprah Winfrey", as Nelson Mandela proclaimed at the school's opening.

Nobel Prize Winner Malala Yousafzai is a fierce equal rights campaigner, on a mission to help the 130 million girls who currently live without access to education. "I think there are hundreds of thousands of Malala's out there," says Yousafzai. "I believe we will see every girl in school in my lifetime." The Malala Fund has raised millions of dollars, which I believe you and I would be very happy about.

Think of some of the wealthiest people in the world, and ask yourself *Am I happy they are wealthy?* Mother Teresa would have been the wealthiest woman on the planet had the world's donations gone into her account and not the Catholic Church's. Personally, I'm very happy that *Exceptionals* like Richard Branson and Michelle Obama (b. 1964) are wealthy. Branson and Obama's commitment to help human beings in need far exceeds their respective professional lives.

If you consider yourself a good person, then wouldn't it be great if you had more money to be good with? Money is nothing more than a magnifier of who you are or consider yourself to be. If you have an exceptional reason or purpose for exceptional wealth, you are far more likely to receive it. If you want to earn $50,000 more or $250,000 more or $20 million more per year, it's important to know the reasons why. If it's simply to buy more shoes or renovate, it's not as likely to happen. Is it so you can send your children to a particular school? Is it so you can buy a family home? Is it so you can start a business? Is it so you can give more to causes you believe in or perhaps even start your own?

If you manage your money wisely, you have exceptional standards as a human being, and you have a great purpose, then I, and billions of other people around the world want you to be financially wealthy!

So what do you choose to be good with?

Once you truly believe that it is a wonderful thing for money to be in your control, you can then turn your attention to identifying the causes that inspire you. What is vital for your exceptional life is choosing causes that stir your heart and soul. In Ikaria, most villages have a festival known as a *panigiri* once per year to commemorate the saint their local church is named after. People from all over the island come together, dining out on bread, tzatziki, Greek salad, goat, hot chips, wine and dessert, dancing the day and night away to live music. In the seaside village of Nas, where the population is around 70, more than 1500 people will attend and raise over 10,000 euro simply by eating and drinking. That money goes towards beautifying the village, repairing roads or paths, or giving to people in need. Having visited Nas regularly since 2016, I notice with joy the physical improvements that are made each year. The path to the beach is improved, safety rails installed, roads have been paved, and families that had medical emergencies have been supported without having to deal with financial hardship on top of everything else.

When you love your community (which is a part of an exceptional social life), finding local causes to contribute to will bring you immense joy. The mantra 'think global, act local' applies as much to your exceptional wealth as it does your environmental behaviour.

The speed of a good cause

A good cause is one that is easy to visualise, making it easy to see your contribution going to good use and invoking hope that your donation will make a difference. I could cite thousands of examples of viral fundraising, however I'm going to share two that are very close to home. They are both on Sarah's side of the family and sadly involve people who eventually died.

Renee was married to Chris, Sarah's brother, and shortly after falling pregnant with their second child, noticed a lump on her kidney. Tests revealed Renee had a rare form of kidney cancer. Shortly after her diagnosis,

Chris and Renee's best friends organised a fundraiser in Melbourne. It was a night of celebration, a fun-filled evening of food, dancing, socialising and good times. When it came to fundraising, the crowd went wild, raising $75,000 in a few short hours.

For more than two years Renee lived with cancer, and the generous gift of donors allowed Renee, Chris, their daughter Grace and soon-to-be-born son, Albi, to have life-treasuring moments. They travelled around Australia, went to theme parks and cherished the time they had. At the age of 39, Renee passed away.

Sarah's niece, Elsie, was two when her parents, Jonny and Jill, noticed a lump in their daughter's abdomen. After a series of tests, Elsie was also diagnosed with a rare form of kidney cancer (Elsie and Renee are not related by blood). Jonny and Jill were naturally stunned at the news, and over the ensuing weeks their family and friends rallied to provide the necessary support. Friends of Jonny and Jill organised a GoFundMe campaign and generated $75,000 in seven days. This took all the pressure off Jonny and Jill to work and they could instead spend quality time with Elsie. The young family spent time in their favourite part of Australia, the Northern Territory, enjoying helicopter rides and some truly unforgettable experiences with their dying daughter. Elsie passed away shortly before her fourth birthday.

Words aren't enough to describe how sad this is that two beautiful souls died so young. When the threat of death looms unexpectedly, we naturally do whatever we can to push it away. The speed by which a community of people will move and take action when a cause is tangible and pulls on the heartstrings is phenomenal.

The more tangible and emotional a cause is to you, the more likely you are to give to it. So consider what *really* gets to you, and top it off by identifying a cause that you can see making a genuine difference.

Leaving Microsoft to change the world

John Wood was an overworked globetrotting Microsoft marketing executive in need of a well-earned break and some fresh air. He chose a hike through the Himalayas of Nepal for his professional convalescence and whilst sipping on a cold beer on his first day in Kathmandu, little did he know that his life was about to change forever. Sitting close by was a local man in his mid-50s named Pasupathi, whose job was to find resources for the local province's 17 schools.

Wood shared with Pasupathi his love of reading as a child and asked about the Nepalese children. Pasupathi invited Wood to a local school for a tour and to meet the students. "I got excited. I was a huge book nerd when I was a kid and I loved school," Wood reflects. "I thought, *this is a chance to see the real Nepal*. So Pasupathi and I set off; we walked about two and a half hours up these very, very steep hills. And we got to this little village called Bahundanda which is where one of his schools was located."[7]

"It was simultaneously hopeful and rather sad. The hopeful bit was that 400 students were showing up every day, eager to learn. Their parents wanted them to learn, but the school was just completely dilapidated. Dirt floors, no ventilation, no natural lighting. You know, 80 kids crammed into a room that should have held not more than 20 kids. And then the children left and the headmaster said, 'Well, let's go see the library.' And I thought, *okay, the library – that will be the hopeful, optimistic part of a tour.*

"We walked into this ramshackle, dirty and dusty room with no light. They had bookshelves but they had no books. And I said to the headmaster, 'How is it you're missing something as important as books in your library for 400 students?' And he said something that would change my life forever. He said, 'Well, in Nepal, we are too poor to afford education but until we have education we will always remain poor.'

"And that struck me as really the kind of the topic sentence of 'why does poverty exist?' Nick Kristof, the *New York Times* writer, one of my favourite writers and a friend has said, 'Talent is universal, opportunity is not.' And I just thought to myself, *this is so sad that 400 kids will grow up, not having the pleasure of reading books. There will be one more generation to be illiterate*. Nepal has one of the highest illiteracy rates in the world. At least it did 20 years ago before we got started with our work. And so the headmaster, like me, was an action-oriented optimist. He gave me a homework assignment. He said, 'Perhaps sir, you will someday come back with books.' And that was a sentence that ultimately would change my life."[8]

Wood not only returned with books, he founded Room to Read, which started as a charity funded by his friends and family and has gone on to distribute over 26 million books to more than 40,000 schools, helping over 20 million children in 15 countries learn to read. Wood's journey to create Room To Read may inspire you to donate to the charity, not because I told you so but because its cause is so great that you feel compelled to do so. Just like Room to Read's story may have inspired you, so should any charitable donation you give your hard-earned money to.

"Without a rich heart wealth is an ugly beggar."
– Ralph Waldo Emerson

▲ ▲ ▲

Creating Exceptional Wealth

Hundreds of thousands of books exist on wealth creation. It's easy to be confused and overwhelmed on the best way to build wealth given that each year a new trend or 'get-rich-quick' scheme comes to life. And whilst it's sensational that we have such easy access to information these days, it does little for our sense of clarity.

I preface this section by saying I come to you in my journalist guise, and not as a financial advisor. Having studied dozens of books on the subject of wealth, I want to do what any good journalist does and provide you with the patterns of financial wisdom that exist in *all* the great books on wealth and wealth creation. For me, here are five books that exist today that I believe are essential reading if you wish to create exceptional wealth.

Think and Grow Rich by Napoleon Hill
How To Make One Hell Of A Profit And Still Get To Heaven by Dr John Demartini
The Richest Man In Babylon by George S. Clason
Money: Master The Game by Tony Robbins
The Barefoot Investor by Scott Pape

You'll find a more in-depth list in the bibliography. The first three books listed apply to anyone in any country at any point in time, whilst Robbins's tome will feel extremely relevant to Americans and Pape's bestseller is definitely published for Australians.

In distilling the wisdom from the greatest books ever written on wealth, all define financial independence the same way. When you have a critical mass of assets and the interest or dividends from those assets provides for your lifestyle, you are financially independent. Put simply, if you have $1 million in assets earning you 8% interest and you can live off $80,000 per year (the interest), you are financially independent and unlikely to ever worry about money again.

To reach financial independence, here are seven principles that, if you genuinely commit to, will yield exceptional wealth relative to your income.

Principle 1: Finance your future by paying yourself first

If the data shows only one thing, it's that spending less than you earn is easier said than done and is most definitely the exception to the rule. The average US household has $16,000 in credit card debt and $30,000 in car loans.[9] Australia has the fourth highest level of household debt in the world, with over 17 million credit cards in circulation and an average debt of over $4000 per card.[10] You've already read in this book that the mantra for exceptional wealth is to 'spend less than you earn and invest the difference'. And whilst this statement is indeed correct, many people do what they can to spend less than they earn without ever paying much attention to 'invest the difference'.

The first decision to make here is *how much* is the difference? George S. Clason's *The Richest Man in Babylon* calls the first cure to a lean purse "Start thy purse to fattening" by keeping at least 10% of your gross income for your future. "For every ten coins thou placest within thy purse take out for use but nine," proclaimed Arkad, the richest man in Babylon.[11] If you are currently like many people and spending over 100% of your income (in other words you have mounting credit card or other bad debt), then your first goal is to get at least $10 for every $100 you earn going into a savings account that is difficult to touch.

If you live without children, have an above-average wage or some other financially favourable circumstances, this savings figure can get to 50% and beyond. Right now, the amount or percentage is not important. The *habit* of routinely placing a set portion of your income aside is the most important financial habit you could ever learn. If this is the only habit of exceptional wealth you ever learn, you're every chance to create financial independence and avoid the catastrophes that many face throughout life and in later years.

Exceptional Exercise 7.1: Pay yourself first

Decide that you will commit to investing the difference – a set amount of your income – no matter how difficult you may find it. Why is saving for your future important to you? Visualise an impoverished future, filled with regret that you spent your years and income on consumables and the demands of today without making tomorrow a priority.

Think of it this way. Break your working week up into 10 half days. The money you earn during your first 'shift' on Monday morning is dedicated to *you and your future*. You are the most important person in your world and your exceptional life demands that you honour this truth immediately.

Principle 2: Cleanse the past by demolishing your debt

Dr John Demartini calls the act of demolishing debt "paying back the people and companies who trusted and invested in you", and I believe that enlightened view makes the process of paying back debt far more fulfilling.

The Barefoot Investor author Scott Pape calls credit cards a 'cult', whilst Positive Real Estate co-founder Jason Whitton (b. 1973) calls them the financial "crack cocaine" of society. "They are the worst thing to financial wellness ever," according to Whitton. "Get off them. If you're on the (financial) ice, if you're on this gear, get off. Even if you pay it off every month, get off it. You know why? Because that's how you (make yourself) feel you are safe. No. Instead, in order to feel safe have $10,000 of savings in your account at any one time. I call it moving the zero line. We react only when our bank account is at zero. You should be reacting when your bank account is at $10,000 going 'something's wrong'. A $10,000 credit card ruins your ability to borrow money by $100,000, even if it's paid off."

With that in mind, timeless wisdom suggests to devote at least 20% of your gross income to *debt demolition*. If, for example, you earn $1000 per week, you are wise to pay $200 per week towards debts, a total of $10,400 per year. If you have $20,000 in credit cards or other bad debts, you know that you will have your debts paid off in approximately two years.

The clarity that this provides is incredibly powerful. If you commit 10% to your future and have bad debts to demolish, you now have 70% of your income to live off. You have clarity, which is more than most people who know they are in debt, but are unsure exactly how much and have no plan to get rid of it.

If this is you right now, I remind you that financial mismanagement does not make you a bad person. Instead, now is the time to own that up until now – for any number of reasons – you haven't given yourself the gift of financial clarity. The time to get your hands dirty and get crystal clear on where you are financially is now. And knowing and owning your level of debt is perhaps the dirtiest your hands will get. This process can be scary and confronting, particularly if you've been racking up debt for some time. However, the power of this newfound clarity, and the commitment to consistently chip away at the debt (and the improved self-esteem this provides) is far more fulfilling.

My personal story of debt

Debt demolition is very close to my heart. Sarah and I were married in 2009 and paid around $40,000 for our wedding. By today's standards that number may be on the lower side of average, but for us, it was the tipping point of our bad debt accrual. Just nine months earlier we had started our own chiropractic business, overcapitalising on equipment we didn't need to buy, racking up debt after debt. I still remember paying over $15,000 for two brand-new, state of the art air compressor chiropractic tables that didn't work properly!

By the time our wedding and honeymoon were complete, we had $55,000 in credit card debt. In Jason Whitton's language, we'd effectively financially overdosed on crack cocaine! Whilst we weren't completely unconscious of our expenditure, the cumulative figure of our debts owing had begun to feel overbearing.

By the end of 2010 our debt had stopped climbing but the interest payable meant we weren't making any inroads. Thankfully, we found a way to consolidate our debts and committed to paying the timeless wisdom number of 20% of our gross income towards debt demolition.

At the time we were paying ourselves $2000 per week from our business. From 2011–2013 we diligently paid $400 per week to debt demolition. When we sold our business in 2013, we had around $14,000 in debt remaining, which we paid off with the proceeds from the sale.

It was three years of discipline, a simple lifestyle (we had young children which made this somewhat easier), and a true recognition of the power of money, but also what true wealth really is. We found that true wealth is more than just money, but that a surplus of money beats debts any day of the week.

During this three-year process we cut up our credit cards and resolved to only ever live on cash. To this day we continue to live without credit cards. We avoid the lure of credit card loyalty programs and enjoy having zero credit card interest hanging over our heads. We live within our means because we've learnt the hard way just what the opposite can do. We are much more disciplined with our cash now than we have ever been, all because of the experiences we went through.

If you can relate to our story, I urge you to focus on what you can gain out of your debt, rather than the pain you have previously or presently experienced. Use that pain as a resource to drive you forward to a place of surplus over deficit. My experience is that paying back debt builds an incredibly strong financial muscle that will serve you forever. Research respectable debt consolidation options and never give up on your quest to have financial independence.

Principle 3: Nourish the now by controlling your expenses

For the ease of this example let's say you've done as above and committed 10% of your gross income to your future and 20% to cleansing the past and demolishing debt. You now have 70% of your income to live off. Because round numbers are easy, let's say you earn $1000 per week. You now have $700 to live off.

Now whilst this may *sound* simple, most people find this very difficult to do, succumbing to increasing debt or stealing from their future (their savings). Keep in mind that 60% of NBA basketballers and 78% of NFL footballers are broke within the first five years after retiring, and they earn above average incomes! So know that this is a test of psychology rather than how much you earn. Whatever your income is, you *can* live within your means, as long as you *believe* you can.

If you're self-employed as I am, it's highly likely your revenue varies week-to-week, month-to-month and year-to-year. In light of this, and upon reading *The Richest Man In Babylon* for the fourth time recently (I tend to read it every two years or so as an audit on my wealth philosophy), a small phrase struck me like never before that applies to us all. Once you've apportioned at least 10% to your future and 20% to your past (if necessary), the secret, according to *The Richest Man in Babylon*, is to then "adjust thy expenditure accordingly". If you earn the same amount each week you are likely to have a great rhythm with this. If your income varies, you are likely to be having some months where some fun and leisurely activities are in the budget and other months they are not.

No matter your income regularity or amount, your responsibility is to be clear on exactly how much you are spending, and what is required to firstly get down to 70% and then live within that amount.

To find out for sure if you are spending less than 70% of your income, a projected budget and your bank statements will give you the answer. The biggest companies in the world set budgets, many of them managing billions of dollars. If it's good enough for them, it's good enough for you and me.

According to Scott Pape in *The Barefoot Investor*: "A good yardstick is allocating 60 per cent of your take-home pay (your after-tax household income) to food, shelter and Netflix – all the things you need to live safely in the suburbs."[12] The other 10% Pape recommends going to a "splurge" account, for the fun and enjoyments of life that you only give yourself when the money is there to enjoy guilt-free.

Pape's rough percentages for expenditure (pull out your calculator) based on average household income are:

> Housing (rent or home loan): 30%
> Utilities (power, gas, water, internet, phone): 5–10%
> Transport: 5–10%
> Insurance: 5%
> Food: 5–10%

Pape's reminder is that this is a guide only and the percentages vary based on income.[13] The challenge is not to let the word 'budget' or the overwhelm of financial clarity stifle your progress to exceptional wealth. "The purpose of a budget is to help thy purse to fatten," reminds *The Richest Man in Babylon*. A budget is not solely for helping us live within our means;

a budget is there to help us achieve financial independence and "realise thy most cherished desires by defending them from thy casual wishes".[14]

> "Wealth consists not in having great possessions,
> but in having few wants."
> – *Epictetus*

Principle 4: Work up the risk ladder

I have been a sucker for 'get-rich-quick' schemes in my life. My twenties was the decade of spending money trying to get rich quick and losing *every single* time. I joined Amway in the hope that I would get rich quickly before heading overseas. I joined another MLM called Dubli and lost close to $10,000 (I should have known better, especially with a name like Dubli). When our daughter Maya was about six months old, I invested in a day-trading course as a way to 'get rich quick' to take the pressure of Sarah working as a chiropractor. That was another $10,000 down the gurgler.

I'm sure you can relate to these three examples from my own life in some small or large way. In each case I ignored the timeless wisdom known as 'working up the risk ladder'. The risk ladder, first explained to me by Dr John Demartini and shared by financial leaders around the globe, forever changed the way I manage my money.

The Risk Ladder

Venture capital or angel investing	High Risk / High Reward
Derivatives (including futures, options and warrants)	
Small-cap stocks	
Mid-cap stocks	Medium Risk / Medium Reward
Large-cap stocks	
Blue Chip stocks	
Bonds	Low Risk / Low Reward
Real Estate	
Index Funds	
Cash	

The least risky financial goal you can start on is to save cash. It's a wise move, creating the discipline of saving 10% of your gross income and letting it sit and accrue interest (no matter how small).

Timeless wisdom suggests to save between 30 and 90 days worth of living expenses as cash and not to use this for investment purposes. The mistake I made in my twenties was to save $10,000 multiple times and skip the more conservative rungs on the risk ladder and blowing it all with a 'get-rich-quick' mentality.

Once you have at least 30 days of living expenses saved, you can begin to look at working up the risk ladder. In this case, it would be an index fund or some government bonds. For decades, investing icon Warren Buffett has recommended investing in index funds. "If you invested in a very low cost index fund, where you don't put the money in at one time, but average in over 10 years, you'll do better than 90% of people who start investing at the same time," says Buffett. "It is not necessary to do extraordinary things to get extraordinary results."

As you work your way up the ladder and continue to invest in chunks of 30 to 90 days, you can begin to invest your money in higher-risk higher-return instruments as your financial and investment knowledge broadens. Many people invest in real estate and do very well there. Others move up to blue chip stocks but don't want to risk investing in mid or small-cap stocks. The game is not about climbing the ladder. The game of wealth is to know your risk threshold and commit to staying at or below it.

The wisdom is to take one rung at a time and only climb the ladder if you choose to – not because you must! Avoid doing as I did in my twenties and jump from the very bottom of the ladder to the very top (investing in derivatives like futures, warrants and options). There is nothing wrong with these more risky strategies, except that they require specialised knowledge and a solid financial base so that you are not putting all of your eggs in one basket.

Despite having heard messages like this from childhood, it has taken me the best part of 20 years to really master and commit to the timeless wisdom of exceptional wealth. My hope for you is that you not only understand the principles in this section but truly begin to action them and make progress in your exceptional wealth, not just for wealth's sake but for the sake of your quality of life and financial independence as you age gracefully.

Having exceptional wealth positively impacts your family life, your health, career, social life and more. If you make the mistake of seeing money as a sign of your status rather than a sign of your inner psychology, you will constantly feel like you are losing or not in possession of enough (as you will always find someone that has more than you).

Using this chapter's example of living on 70% of your income ($700 each week), your first investment goal is to save 90 days of living expenses (13 weeks), a total of $9100. When you do, you won't go to bed at night worried about money or a roof over your head. Then, and only then, do you give yourself permission to begin saving for an investment on the next rung of the investment ladder, real estate or index funds. Start at the beginning, climb the ladder one rung at a time and avoid the temptation to skip ahead.

> *"Rule No. 1 is never lose money.*
> *Rule No. 2 is never forget Rule No. 1."*
> *– Warren Buffett*

Principle 5: Know your numbers

I read *Rich Dad Poor Dad* by Robert Kiyosaki when I was 19 and was inspired to get clarity on my personal finances. At that stage of my life I had very little financial literacy, and Kiyosaki's bestseller was both confronting and eye-opening.

If you were a business on the stock market or a business for sale, would you be an attractive buy? If you say "absolutely not" or "I have no idea", it's likely to be because you have no awareness of your balance sheet or you know it's terrible. So, how do you find this clarity? *Rich Dad Poor Dad* and countless other financial texts refer to four key figures that will make it clear whether you are in healthy or unhealthy financial shape.

1. Your total assets
2. Your total liabilities
3. Your income
4. Your expenses

This exercise could take as little as five minutes if you're organised or 30 days if you have your financial information fragmented across multiple accountants, superannuation funds, shoeboxes and bank accounts. No matter how long it takes, the time is a small price to pay for the clarity on where you currently are financially. You must know where you *are* before determining where you want to go. Identifying the value of your assets, liabilities, income and expenses will show you where you are financially right now.

Exceptional Exercise 7.2: Know your cashflow position

Draw a four-column table or write in the spaces below your sources of income and amounts and your total expenses. If you followed principle 3 you ideally already know your annual expenses.

Income source	Amount (gross)	Expenses	Amount (gross)
Salary	$52,000	Annual	$50,000

My cashflow position as of today (total income minus expenses) =

$_____

Exceptional Exercise 7.3: Know your financial net worth

To discover your financial net worth you'll need an inventory of your assets and your liabilities. Assets may include cash on hand, home contents, superannuation, stocks, real estate, motor vehicles and more. Liabilities most typically are any loans you have to a third party of any kind (and yes, that includes family loans if you have them).

Assets		Liabilities	
Equity in home (The value of your home minus the mortgage you owe)	$	Home loan (The amount you owe the lender)	$
Contents	$	Credit cards	$
Cash	$	Education loans	$
Stocks	$	Car loan	$
Superannuation	$	Personal loan	$
Equity in investment properties	$	Investment property loans	$
Total		**Total**	

My net worth as of today (assets total minus liabilities total) =

$_____

Principle 6: Have a vision for your wealth

The faster the world moves the harder it seems to be for people to think more than a year or two in advance. The brutal financial reality is that most people will be on government welfare when they retire. More than two-thirds of Australians are on the age pension, and as people get older (and they run out of money), that number rises to more than 80%.[15]

Given that it's highly likely you'll be alive at retirement age, I have no doubt you'd prefer to avoid relative poverty and end up on the age pension. My suggestion is to aim for financial independence, relative to your lifestyle needs. Statistically, the odds are stacked against you, which means you have to really want exceptional wealth in order to create it. However, if you follow the principles outlined in this book by some of the masters of wealth, financial independence is yours for the taking.

Remember, the major reason why people fall in to the age pension is their lack of vision. When you have a vision for your wealth, and commit to it for at least 20 years, it's highly likely you'll end up wealthy.

When you complete the following exercise, the numbers might frighten you. If that's the case, harness that fear into the creation of a vision for your financial future, and then seek the support you need in order to make it happen. If you don't have a vision for your wealth and stick to it, financial mediocrity and relative poverty is your only option.[16]

Exceptional Exercise 7.4: Know your financial independence number

The following exercise was first taught to me in 2011 by Dr John Demartini at his *Prophecy I* seven-day workshop in Sydney. If you're anything like me, when you complete this exercise for the first time, the numbers may frighten you. This fear is perhaps why most people never create exceptional wealth. For me – and hopefully you – this exercise was the catalyst to seriously commit to improving my financial health.

Step 1: Get yourself a piece of paper and in the middle at the top of the page write down what it costs you to live each year. For ease of numbers in this example I'm going to say $50,000.

Step 2: Below this number write what your dream lifestyle would cost each year. Let's say it's $150,000.

Step 3: Dr Demartini taught me the wisdom of striking a balance between the optimist and the pessimist (I'm a raging optimist as you may have gathered), so now add these two figures together and divide by two. In my example $50,000 + $150,000 divided by two brings an average cost of living to $100,000.

Step 4: Now here's where it gets interesting and real. Depending on your age and financial health right now, this average cost of living could be closer or further away from your reality than you think. Write down your age as of today (my example is 40) and make an indent across the page in 15-year increments until you reach 100. Don't assume you'll die before you blow out 100 candles on the cake. Again, conservatism and the long view is wiser than reckless 'get-rich-quick' abandon when it comes to creating exceptional wealth.

Under today's age, write down your averaged cost of living. In my example, $100,000. At each 15-year increment double the amount. My example would look like this.

40	55	70	85	100
$100,000	$200,000	$400,000	$800,000	$1,600,000

Dr Demartini shared with me that the reason he uses 15-year increments is due to the average rate of inflation over the last 100 years (which is 4.8%). Using the financial principle known as the Rule of 72, when you divide 72 by 4.8% you get a doubling rate of 15.[17] In other words, the cost of living is likely to double every 15 years. From ice cream to real estate, this number stacks up against almost anything.

Looking at your numbers, you may find your heart begin to flutter somewhat when you look at the income you'll need at age 85 or 100 just to live the same way you do today. A quick glance at history will show you that these numbers aren't at all fanciful. More importantly, you and I are unlikely to be exchanging our time for money when we're 85 or 100 – so where is the money going to come from? As previously mentioned, you don't want to be relying on government welfare to sustain your lifestyle, and you don't want to be dependent on children and friends to give you money to live.

Step 5: Exceptional wealth means that you have other sources of income outside of a job to fund your lifestyle. To find out exactly what this amount is, Dr Demartini taught me the average interest on savings and investments averages 8% per year, approximately one twelfth of the asset. To "know your number", multiply your cost of living by 12 and that is the amount of assets you need to own *outright* to live the lifestyle you want. In my example of having a $100,000 lifestyle at age 40, I would need to own outright assets to the value of $1.2 million. When I blow 100 candles out on the cake, I'll need to have $19.2 million in assets, generating an 8% return, providing for my lifestyle which will cost $1.6 million each year.

Step 6: Looking at your own numbers now, ask yourself if you're on track or not? Don't beat yourself up if you're wildly off track. I can tell you that most people who end up on the pension were so far off track without knowing it because they *never knew their number*. You now know your number. The question is, what are you going to do with it? Maybe you're on track and it's a matter of staying the course. If you're off track, are you going to give up before you even start? Or, are you now going to adjust your entire belief system about saving, spending and investing the money you work so hard to bring in to your life.

Most importantly, use this financial future exercise to consider every element of your exceptional life. What happens in every other area of life if you don't create financial independence? How will it impact your children's life? If you end up on welfare will that cause significant stress to your family and friends? Would it impact where you live, and as a result who you hang around? Would your food choices be impacted by being on welfare, and thereby put you at risk of disease? Would poor financial wealth impact your ability to visit family in far-away destinations? Would you not see the children or grandchildren as often because you couldn't afford the airfares? Is it possible poor financial health may even prevent you from attending the funerals of old friends? And is it possible that being financially broke may negatively impact your world view and faith in humanity?

Whilst money is not the secret to happiness, wealth – in all its definitions – has infinite potential to colour your years with a brightness that nothing else can.

Principle 7: In order to earn more, learn more

With no doubt bigger numbers than you ever thought now swirling around you, you may be thinking how you will create an income that will help you meet your goals. Personally I am far more inclined to focus on how I can grow my income more than reduce my expenses. It is far more exciting and thrilling for me to focus on adding value to society and being rewarded for it rather than continually crunching my lifestyle.

Whilst it's essential to know what your expenses are, at some point you will know how much it costs to run You Inc or Your Family Inc and you'll find there's only so much you can screw down on your expenses.

Once you master your expenses you are likely to reach a point where it's time to focus on income. And one of the most fulfilling ways to earn more is to learn more. Whether you're an employee or business-owner, up-skilling is often the key to adding either another stream of income or improving your income.

The question is, what do *you want* to learn that is valuable to the marketplace? Importantly, what you choose to learn must inspire you. It can't be something that is *only* good for the marketplace, but dead boring and uninspiring to you. You will run out of steam and end up resenting the time, effort and money you put in to the study.

You may want to learn Mandarin so that you can travel to China and do business more easily. You may want to get an MBA to make career advancement more likely. You may be an incredible parent who loves business and decide to open childcare centres. You may be a carpenter who wants to become a builder. You may be learning about property investment or stocks, developing your speaking skills or mastering the online marketing world of blogs, social media and selling products and services online.

A great question to ask yourself is: *What do I want to learn more of that will allow me to earn more?*

Remember, the key word is what do you *want* to learn; not what do you *need* to learn or *have* to learn. Human beings learn most effortlessly when they are inspired to learn. If other people are telling you to learn something, be sure to ask yourself if it's important to you.

Alternatively, you may decide an amount of income you want to earn over the year or next few years and then write down all the missing knowledge required to learn by you (or others) in order to get that result. In either approach, behaving out of inspiration over desperation will guarantee longevity in your pursuit of exceptional wealth.

> *"Formal education will make you a living;*
> *self-education will make you a fortune."*
> *– Jim Rohn*

Give with warm hands

"My father used to say to me when I was eight years old. 'Eddie, there's more pleasure in giving than taking.' I thought he was cuckoo. Now that I have children and grandchildren and great grandchildren I like to give with warm hands. My children won't have to wait until I die (to receive my money). I like to see what they do with the money. This is giving me more pleasure to enjoy my own money by giving it now so that I can see what happens with this money."

– **Eddie Jaku OAM, Holocaust survivor and author of** *The Happiest Man On Earth.*

PART THREE

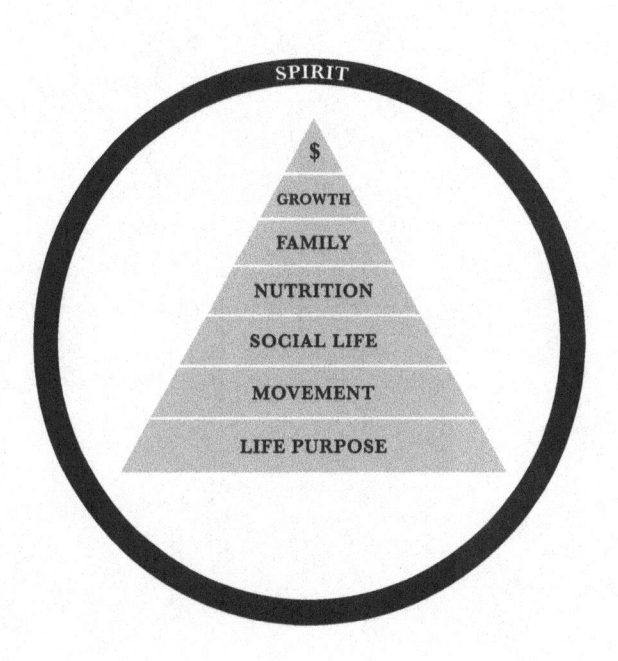

YOUR EXCEPTIONAL
SPIRIT

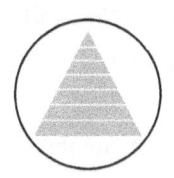

SPIRIT

> "Out beyond ideas of wrongdoing and rightdoing,
> there is a field. I'll meet you there."
> *– Rumi*

In something as seemingly abstract as spirit, there is a clear defining line between *The Exceptionals* and the rest of society. *The Exceptionals* fully express their great spirit. The rest of us are too scared to. *The Exceptionals* live with a resounding spirit in the tough times as well as the good times. The rest of us play the victim. *The Exceptionals* are always looking at how to be the victor, no matter how great the adversity.

From Turia Pitt having two-thirds of her body burnt to Helen Keller being deaf and blind and still graduating from Harvard. Yes, *The Exceptionals* seem to suffer more than most, and perhaps those challenges create immense spiritual muscle.

But it's not only adversity that builds an exceptional spirit. *The Exceptionals* find a way to navigate and spiritually profit from a world littered with opposing forces – love and hate, wealth and poverty, war and peace among them. The exceptional spirit finds immense purpose in the dualities of life rather than ride its alluring rollercoaster of euphoric highs and depressive lows. In fact, many of *The Exceptionals* we know and love wouldn't exist if it wasn't for the opposing problem they were trying to solve. No Mandela without apartheid. No Mother Teresa without poverty. No Malala without the Taliban. Indeed, *The Exceptionals* see that problems provide purpose.

And just as we begin to appreciate the gift of these opposites in conflict, the ego, in a last-ditch attempt to remain alive, throws soul-limiting grenades at us in the form of expectations, fear and judgement that make it impossible to fully express ourselves if we give up. But *The Exceptionals* never, ever give up. *The Exceptionals* conquer immense pain and adversity. *The Exceptionals* transcend a world built on opposing forces. *The Exceptionals* defy the safety-enhancing lure of judgement, fear and expectation. *The Exceptionals* go for the spiritual jugular – often by way of a faith-based spiritual practice bedded in prayer and gratitude, laid down on a strong yet simple foundation of sleep and breath that allows our body to fully express the limitless soul that we are.

▲ ▲ ▲

Putting Your Spirit Into Every Area of Life

I've worked with thousands of men and women who make it extremely difficult for themselves to feel good. They are often excelling in many areas of life, yet they have made the art of spiritual fulfilment an unattainable masterpiece. 'Everything' needs to go right in order to be happy. All items on the daily to-do list must be ticked off. Happiness exists only when a certain amount of money is in the bank, the house is paid off, or the business has hit a particular milestone. This impossible path to happiness is fuelled by the ego, filled with labels of good and bad, right and wrong, success and failure.

The ego is defined by the *Oxford Dictionary* as: "a person's sense of self-esteem or self-importance". Your spirit is not interested in either. Your spirit is "the non-physical part of a person which is the seat of emotions and character; the soul". When you bake a cake that doesn't rise, your ego admonishes you, whilst your soul remains still. When you yell at your children or partner your ego lowers your self-esteem whilst your soul loves you no matter what. When you achieve a goal your ego bursts with pride whilst your soul remains calm and unchanged. Said another way, the ego fluctuates in the bell curve of life's 'good' and 'bad' experiences, punishing you in the bad times and jumping on the bandwagon in the good times. Your spirit, meanwhile, is with you forever, unconditionally tied to every experience of your life.

It's your spirit that gets you up early or stays up late to complete a project; it's your spirit that completes an extra push up or gets up at 5am to walk in the dark; it's your spirit that gets you through grieving for friends or family no longer here; it's your spirit that delivers a vision for your financial future. Without your spirit, your exceptional life can descend into a bunch of to-do lists, reduced to the uninspiring world of administration and jobs. Your romantic relationship atrophies into a combination of text messages and quick phone calls, your work becomes one big email train, your nutrition an overwhelming meal plan and your financial future a cornucopia of transactions on a bank statement. The exceptional life that you are living feels anything but, consumed with everything you need to 'get done' and still feeling like a failure when you do achieve your goals.

And so let us now infuse the final ingredient into the recipe called *Your Exceptional Life*. This is an ingredient unlike any of the preceding seven. It's not one that you can measure simply in isolation like you can with movement or nutrition. Instead, your spirit is something which can only be measured when it's included and observed in each area of life. If you hold back from putting your spirit into all you do, you'll find a distinct lack of fulfilment that the feeling of comfort won't tell you about until it has well and truly arrived in the form of regret.

Making the abstract and esoteric concrete and practical

The conversation around spirituality often contains esoteric and abstract language, leaving many people timid or confused. Whilst I have great respect for the untouchable and invisible, I want to focus this section on unleashing your exceptional spirit through a practical step-by-step process.

In order to put our heart and soul into each area of life, there are four lessons we must all learn for our exceptional spirit to flourish.

Firstly, it is without doubt that all human beings experience significant pain of some type. We might say that 'bad' things happen to 'good' people. Now whilst the spirit doesn't label events and people as good or bad, there seems to be no getting around the human experience of pain.

Secondly, as Jim Rohn once outlined: "Opposites are in conflict and we are in the middle." Our spirit has an easier time expressing itself when we accept and appreciate that we can only define peace because of war, that love cannot exist without hate, that light is an absence of darkness and so on.

Thirdly, after all is said and done, an exceptional spirit sees beyond the first two limitations. Whilst this may require significant pain and a prolonged exposure to the two sides of life, the first two lessons leave *The Exceptionals* without any doubt that the soul is limitless, and an awareness of this is required to live a life of spiritual fulfilment.

Finally, when the rubber hits the road there are many spiritual practices to choose from. From the day we are born to the day we die, we are as the saying goes, 'spiritual beings having a human experience' and not 'human beings having a spiritual experience.' The sooner you decide to live by this mantra and consciously incorporate your spirit into your daily life, the sooner you'll experience the full range of blessings available to you.

▲ ▲ ▲

Lesson 1: Pain is Inevitable

Eddie Jaku still can't understand how his countrymen murdered his family during the Holocaust. Turia Pitt still lives with the pain of two-thirds of her body being burnt in 2011. Malala Yousafzai still endures the effects of being shot in the head by the Taliban when she was 15. Stephen Hawking (1942–2018) was diagnosed with Motor Neurone Disease at age 21, given two years to live and died 55 years later. For any number of reasons it seems *The Exceptionals* live with more than their fair share of heartache and pain, and it's their seemingly impossible recovery from adversity that often makes them inspiring.

It's not that *The Exceptionals* have 'better' souls, for we are all *Exceptionals*. Instead, the only feature distinguishing *The Exceptionals* from the rest of society is attitude. An exceptional makes the most of any circumstance and lives with a can-do attitude despite the harshest of cards being dealt. Any war veteran, genocide survivor or displaced human being could quite easily be forgiven for succumbing to the ravages of mediocrity. Many have, and yet there are also countless inspirations who have chosen an empowering attitude to life instead.

Between what happens to us and how we respond lives a space that houses our exceptional life. In that space is our thoughts and beliefs that dictate our response to any event. Our perspective of what happens to us in life shapes our response to each event and eventually our entire life.

The response most people create is to be a victim of circumstance. We human beings love to play the victim. It's a safe, socially accepted, sympathy-inducing form of behaviour that entails 'bad' things happening 'to' you, with no positive consequences or blessings in disguise. I'm not referring to victims who die unsavoury deaths; I'm referring to 'victims' who live, and perpetuate a victim story for the rest of their life. Whilst *The Exceptionals* undoubtedly go through phases of victim thinking, they grow through this phase to find the hidden order in their experiences.

Take grief for example. The 5 Stages of Grief®, first created by Swiss psychiatrist Elisabeth Kübler-Ross outlines the path of grieving as one of denial, anger, bargaining, depression and finally acceptance.[1]

If one never fully accepts the death of the person they're grieving, they are stuck in denial, anger, depression, or living with a constant internal bargaining (such as "it should have been me instead"), all of which entail victim thinking. Our job is not to blame the grieving person (especially if it's ourselves) for being stuck in one of the first four phases. Instead, our role is to understand that acceptance is the 'exceptional' phase of grief that we are permitted and entitled to experience.

There are countless inspiring examples of people who have had their spirits seemingly broken and gone on to use their experiences to their greatest advantage and lived extraordinary lives. And it's these people – the ones who lead by example and progress past being a victim – who generally inspire us the most.

It's what American professor Joseph Campbell referred to as 'The Hero's Journey'. No matter what you call it, a great spiritual transformation takes place amidst remarkable challenge where one goes from victim to victor. Helen Keller's (1880–1968) achievements and message wouldn't be anywhere near as inspiring to us if she hadn't suffered the afflictions of deafness and blindness. Turia Pitt is a hero to millions *because* of the trauma she experienced and the victim-free attitude she has chosen to have. "We all have that inner strength inside of us, but we just never get tested. So we never get the chance to discover how incredible we all are," Pitt reflected in 2014, three years after enduring burns to 65% of her body.[2]

What makes Nelson Mandela so inspiring is that he overcame so many hurdles and refused to play the victim. "Difficulties break some men but make others," wrote Mandela in 1975 in a letter to his wife Winnie whilst imprisoned on Robben Island. "No axe is sharp enough to cut the soul of a sinner who keeps on trying, one armed with the hope that he will rise even in the end." In the midst of your inevitable pain is the decision that must be made: will you succumb to the difficulties and let the axe cut your soul?

> *"We could never learn to be brave and patient if there were only joy in the world."*
> *– Helen Keller*

Create your own challenges

If you haven't experienced the tragic trauma of Nelson Mandela's life and expect you will never get close to that type of hardship, it's only natural that you're likely to avoid significant challenge and difficulty on a daily basis. Human beings are not naturally wired for hardship, so we need to consciously create it, given the modern comforts that many of us now live with. As counterintuitive as it may sound – if you have lived, as I have, without major trauma in your life (by 'major' I mean the type of trauma the news would report), it's more important than ever to make life that little bit more challenging.

Creating your own challenges might be quitting a job you hate or starting the business you've always dreamed of but been too scared to start. In your movement it might be running a marathon or simply parking the car some distance from the supermarket and walking back holding heavy bags. Socially it might be mustering the courage to end the friendship that served you during school but doesn't 20 years later. Nutritionally it could be eliminating or heavily reducing white sugar and gluten. In your family life it may be ditching Netflix at night and having meaningful conversations and experiences with your loved ones. Learning a language or studying a new skill may be a challenge you actively create in your growth, whilst your wealth challenge may be to test your discipline by saving a minimum 10% of your gross income from this day forward.

If instead you opt for the path of least resistance and chronic comfort, you risk your final years engulfed by the eight consequences of mediocrity – regret, cognitive decline, depression, disease, bitterness, boredom, financially broke and spiritually broken.

Transforming pessimism and pain into learned or tragic optimism

The inconvenient truth is that some people have far more traumatic lives than others. Some experience the trauma of war, poverty and murder, burying multiple children and family members over the course of their lives. Others go through life never burying a child, and at worst lose their parents to cancer, heart disease or dementia.

But that doesn't make spiritual heartache exclusively reserved for the most tragic cases. Miscarriages, suicides, drug problems and domestic violence are just some of the sources of significant challenges people face every day that won't make the news headlines.

Regardless of the amount of tragedy you've personally encountered, you will have an optimistic or pessimistic view of your experiences and the world around you. Viktor Frankl (1905–1997), author of *Man's Search For Meaning*, termed his own optimism and the optimism of anyone who had endured significant heartache as a "tragic optimism". His theory of logotherapy, which by definition is "a conviction that the primary human drive is not pleasure but the pursuit of what we find meaningful," maintains that optimism can still take place in spite of what he calls the "tragic triad" – pain, guilt and death.

"What matters is to make the best of any given situation," Frankl writes. "A tragic optimism, that is, an optimism in the face of tragedy and in view of the human potential which at its best always allows for: (1) turning suffering into a human achievement and accomplishment; (2) deriving from guilt the opportunity to change oneself for the better; and (3) deriving from life's transitoriness an incentive to take responsible action."[3]

So there you have your challenge to live your exceptional life. To paraphrase Frankl, will you turn your suffering into an accomplishment and achievement? Will you view your guilt as an opportunity to improve yourself and your life? And will you acknowledge that your inevitable death provides you with an opportunity to write the script of your life and follow your heart's desires? You don't need to experience Auschwitz to make these decisions. Millions of people like Frankl have suffered on our behalf; our *obligation* as fellow human beings is to honour their experiences by living our own exceptional life.

Frankl maintains that optimism cannot be "commanded or ordered. One cannot even force oneself to be optimistic indiscriminately, against all odds, against all hope. And what is true for hope is also true for the other two components of the triad inasmuch as faith and love cannot be commanded or ordered either."[4]

Optimism can be learned

As American psychologist Martin Seligman demonstrates in his groundbreaking books *Learned Optimism* and *Learned Helplessness*, optimism is available to all of us. Seligman argues that whilst we can't control what happens to us, we can control the explanation or story we tell (and thereby our levels of optimism). The pessimist reading this book is likely to resist this notion just as much as an optimist would resist the idea that they could become pessimistic.

For the sake of allowing your spirit to soar and finding meaning in your life's toughest times, knowing whether you're currently an optimist or pessimist is pivotal, particularly if you're the latter. Seligman's work centres on the particular traits of pessimists and optimists. A pessimist believes bad events will last a long time, will impact much of what they do, and sometimes blame themselves or inappropriately take responsibility. Given the same set of bad events, optimists view them as road works rather than road closures, in other words as isolated incidents. Losses are not their fault, with a dose of bad luck, fate or someone else often the reason. Optimists are more likely to push on during tough times, whereas pessimists are more inclined to give up.

So where do you sit? Are you an optimist or a pessimist? And if you are a pessimist, are you prepared to practise optimism to the point where it becomes learned behaviour? If you are, Seligman's chief recommendation is to practise the art of relentlessly disputing your pessimistic beliefs. For example, if you start hating on yourself, ask yourself genuinely if what you are saying is true. If you believe it is, then work on the solution rather than the problem. For example, if you believe you're a terrible spouse, friend or colleague, how can you alter this?

Yet Seligman believes that most of the time our negative beliefs are distortions, with the best response to challenge those beliefs and stop them from running our life. And reassuringly, learned optimism is a healthy addiction and easy to maintain once the muscle has been developed. For the learned optimist, life becomes somewhat smoother, happiness easier to experience, and resilience easier to develop.

Whether you practise Frankl's tragic optimism, Seligman's learned optimism or your own born optimism, all require a can-do attitude to apply an empowering meaning to the inevitable pain and challenge you'll experience in life. When you begin to control your thoughts in this way, you become as the poet William Henley proclaimed in his stoic poem 'Invictus'; the master of your fate and the captain of your soul.

> Out of the night that covers me
> Black as the pit from pole to pole,
> I thank whatever gods may be
> For my unconquerable soul.
>
> In the fell clutch of circumstance,
> I have not winced nor cried aloud.
> Under the bludgeonings of chance
> My head is bloody, but unbowed.
>
> Beyond this place of wrath and tears
> Looms but the Horror of the shade,
> And yet the menace of the years
> Finds, and shall find, me unafraid.
>
> It matters not how strait the gate,
> How charged with punishments the scroll,
> I am the master of my fate:
> I am the captain of my soul.

– 'Invictus' by William Henley

▲ ▲ ▲

Lesson 2: We Live in a Conflict of Opposites

Regardless of how optimistic or pessimistic you are, both traits will always exist within you. "It seems like opposites are in conflict and we are in the middle," expressed speaker and author Jim Rohn. "Evil on one side; good on the other. Illness on one side; good health on the other. Darkness on one side; light on the other."

The challenge we face over the course of our exceptional life is to accept and appreciate both sides of life, and to accept our position 'in the middle'.

Whilst *The Exceptionals* either innately or through their life experiences master the art of living 'in the middle', most in society firmly attach themselves to one-sided beliefs, character traits and outcomes. I for one spent years attempting to be constantly happy and never sad, always positive and never negative, always can-do and never can't-do – and I expected others to be the same way. It's easy to expect your partner and friends to support you at all times, to crave world peace and refute war, to bemoan disease and strive for wellness. As socially acceptable – and even encouraged – as all of this may be, it's a gross mistake to expect to live a one-sided life. Sooner or later (and hopefully sooner so the lesson can be learnt), we get brought back to the middle by way of the 'other side' drawing us in.

I've already shared the fate of diet experts who died prematurely from sickness. There are countless cases of everyday wellness enthusiasts who ate the perfect diet, did yoga and meditated every morning, and developed a chronic disease. There are also millions of people-pleasers who 'support' and 'love' everyone outwardly and experience an overwhelming undercurrent of resentment and self-hate on the inside. The more we attempt to remove one side of our life experience the more it seems to come back to haunt us.

No matter how hard we try to stop it, we will never have world peace without war going on somewhere on the planet. There will never be true love without true hate happening somewhere else. And whilst you might experience the peak of health, someone else is going through the trough of sickness. Our challenge is to see these conflicts of opposites as heaven on earth, and bask in our time here as spiritual beings having a 'human experience'.

Conflict of Opposites 1: Happiness and sadness

It's likely that your problem is not that you aren't happy all the time, but instead that you are not letting yourself be happier. This is endemic in people who focus solely on results whilst forgetting to enjoy the journey or adventure of life. Statements starting with 'I'll be happy when' are a shortcut to sadness, frustration and anger.

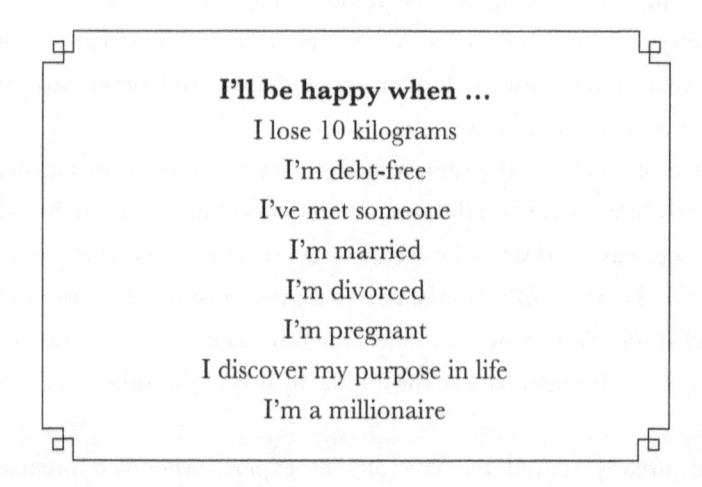

> **I'll be happy when ...**
> I lose 10 kilograms
> I'm debt-free
> I've met someone
> I'm married
> I'm divorced
> I'm pregnant
> I discover my purpose in life
> I'm a millionaire

Such limiting beliefs close the window on happiness so that even the celebration of victory is muted. If, in fact, we do celebrate, we hastily 'move on' to the next project or goal, unknowingly putting at risk a deeper fulfilment that becomes unattainable and is often replaced by regret at the end of our lives.

"We all have a positive contribution to make. I've made mine," reflected 51-year-old Cath whilst lying on her deathbed. "But while I was searching for my purpose in life, I forgot to enjoy myself along the way. It was all about the result of finding what I was looking for. Then when I did find work I loved, work I could do with the heartfelt intention of contributing, I was still results-based."[5]

Cath's story, detailed in Bronnie Ware's *The Top Five Regrets of the Dying* is equal parts heart-breaking and spiritually resuscitating. "I have robbed myself of potential happiness. It is important, sure, to work towards finding your purpose and contributing to the world, in any capacity. But depending on the end result for your happiness is not the way to do it."[6]

If you're on the other team, the effervescently positive 'happy all the time' camp, you're easily forgiven. A quick Google, Amazon or social media search will return a swathe of 'happy all the time' memes, books and quotes that conveniently forget to address the important role sadness plays in our lives.

Your sadness shows your truth as much as your happiness does. Take grief for example. It's completely natural and normal to be overcome with sadness at the loss of a loved one. However, many cultures today encourage us to move on with a certain stoicicism that if we fail to adopt, we're seen as emotionally weak and in need of medication to get us back to 'normal'.

"We tend to overmedicate for depression," neuropsychologist Dr Mario Martinez shared with me on *100 Not Out*. "People are not allowed to mourn death or the end of a relationship. They are not allowed to express emotions other than happy, so we get overmedicated." Whilst it may sound flippant, the statistics show something else. At the time of going to print, almost 10% of the world's population is on antidepressants, with Iceland, Australia, Canada and the United Kingdom the planet's highest consumers.[7] During the COVID-19 ravaged 2020, antidepressant sales were expected to double from US $14.3 billion in 2019 to $28.6 billion just 12 months later.[8]

Conflict of Opposites 2: Love and hate

Much has been spoken about love and hate already, particularly in the section on family. Many people have difficulty with the word 'hate' as it's almost counterintuitive (and perhaps goes against our better judgement) to admit that we hate something or someone.

At the same time, there are many people who hate cancer, hate death, hate governments, hate the rain, hate kale, hate traffic, hate perpetrators of crimes and hate family members. So as much as it may seem cruel to hate, it's not uncommon.

You may actually need to 'hate' some part of your life in order to improve it. Hate may be too strong a word for you, so you may use the word 'can't stand' or 'mediocre' or 'healthy discontent' instead. Take your intimate relationship status for example. You have to feel that it is 'average' or 'empty' or 'painful' in order for you to improve it. Even if it's exceptional right now, you need to believe that doing nothing to maintain a great relationship will create pain. In other words, you need to hate mediocrity.

At the same time, and at risk of being confusing, you also need to *love* hate for what it shows you about yourself. Hate is the cue for change. Hate is the cue for transformation. It is the subtle whisper or the ear-splitting scream demanding you to grow. Hate challenges you to truly love in the most unconditional way.

To remove hate of other people, we must come to the conclusion that the hate is holding us back or preventing us from receiving something we want. As *Schindler's List* Holocaust survivor Celina Biniaz (b. 1931) explains to secondary school children: "I'm pushing forward the idea that you have to get rid of any kind of hatred because hatred is corrosive," Biniaz shared with me on *100 Not Out*. "A lot of people not only respond to my background because of what I went through but they are impressed that I was able to work my way through it and continue to have a decent life and even though they may have issues at home, the idea is to work through those issues to be able to move forward in your life."

Are you doing the work on your own corrosive hatred so that you can move forward in your life? If not, the inevitable emptiness, resentment and regret at avoiding the deeper work finds a way of insidiously impacting all the areas of life you worked to make exceptional. The key to avoiding this undesirable fate is to unpack *who* or *what* you hate, *how* you hate and *why* you hate.

Exceptional Exercise 8.1:
The Who, What, Why and How of Hate

Who or what do you hate?	How do you hate?	Why do you hate?
Traffic	Anger	Makes me late to work, I have better things to do
My brother	Avoidance and excluding him from family events	He coerced Mum and Dad to have the will made in his favour
Political leader of my country	Talk and think about them with disdain or venom	Where do I start? Bigoted, corrupt, sociopath

Once you have completed this exercise, consider ways in which you could love or appreciate the thing or person you hate. What empowering meaning could you put on the events that have taken place in your life? What potential opportunity is your hatred presenting you with? If this is triggering you, use the methods outlined in the forgiveness section of family to help forgive and accept.

Conflict of Opposites 3: Sickness and health

Our world-view can change overnight by seeing people we love die for what looks like unjust reasons. Why did that healthy person die from cancer, when the neighbour down the road who smokes a packet of cigarettes each day is still fighting fit?

What we must recognise, and hopefully you have gleaned through reading this book, is that life is far more complex than 'you are what you eat', 'smoking will kill you' and 'family comes first'. Cancer can start in the womb, years before a child is even diagnosed.[9] Why does cancer even exist? That's a topic for an entirely different book, but like every challenge in life, diseases and sickness are here to teach us and help us grow in life – if we're prepared to listen and learn.

Let me now share with you my brother-in-law Chris's experience following the passing of his wife, Renee, who died of cancer aged 39. Chris and Renee had always wanted to move to Byron Bay. They were engaged there and had often dreamt of relocating to Australia's most easterly town. With the majority of family and friends in Victoria and their daughter, Grace, in school, combined with the pressures of daily life (not to mention the many challenges of moving interstate), they never moved to Byron Bay.

Enter cancer of the kidney.

In the 28 months from diagnosis to death, Chris and Renee had their second child, Albi, went on multiple trips around Australia (including a visit to Byron Bay) and did many things they'd always wanted to do, but had never got around to. Chris nursed his wife the entire time with an unconditional love that was inspirational to observe.

When Renee died, you can imagine the turmoil. But in the light of day, Chris – heartbroken and grieving – was philosophical, saying: "Renee lived her life's purpose. What she wanted most in life was to have children and enjoy her family. She was content; she was fulfilled. She did what she came here to do. We all want her back; I miss her every day; but her leaving taught me so much about life."

Within six months of Renee dying, Chris made one of the biggest decisions of his life – to move to Byron Bay. "The choice was clear; I could either regret for the rest of my life that we never did it whilst Renee was alive, or I could give myself and our children the lifestyle that Renee and I had always dreamt of having."

In a further twist, Chris's brother Ash and his family also decided to move to the Byron Shire. By January 2017 the three Martin siblings – Sarah (my wife), Chris and Ash all lived within a short drive from each other. And in a heartwarming completion of the story, by the end of 2019, their parents Rob and Jill made the big move too.

The legacy of Renee's 39 years on earth continues to affect more than just her immediate family. The entire Martin lineage owes part of their everyday experience to the life of Renee. Her death planted the tree that she'll never sit under: grandparents watching their adult children and grandchildren grow up together, cousins growing up together, going to school together, camping together, fishing together, having sleepovers together and celebrating birthdays together. Just as I wouldn't be alive if it weren't for the death of Annie Seymour, it's unlikely the Martin family would have the proximity and multi-generational connectedness if it weren't for Renee's death.

Often our greatest sadness is laced with the seeds of great opportunity and future joy. It's only the passage of time that uncovers the hidden wonder and benefit of sickness and disease, whilst making us incredibly grateful for the gift of good health.

Conflict of Opposites 4: Birth and death

Most people see birth as a time to celebrate and death as a time to commiserate. No one ever grieves that a newborn baby will eventually die, despite every single one of us being born with the 'terminal illness' of death.

Our extreme avoidance of death and desperate attempt to cling to our youth causes many of us to forget to enjoy the days, weeks, months, years and decades we all potentially have on this planet. In our childhood we are often asked what we want to be when we grow up and then as we grow up we grieve our lost youth and fear our mortality. We rarely seem comfortable in the here and now. As Eckhart Tolle expresses in *The Power of Now: A Guide to Spiritual Enlightenment*, our future-based thinking generates anxiety and our past-based thinking generates guilt. It's only in the 'now' that we can experience true presence.

Rohn's view that we are 'caught in the middle' of a conflict of opposites – in this case birth and death – is in fact what the gift of life truly is. We need birth *and* death in order to have life itself. The fact that life ends provides us all with a spiritual urgency and opportunity to live each day as if it's the final one. This doesn't mean we go skydiving and jump off cliffs every day; it means we live simply but powerfully, as outlined throughout this book.

Said another way, can you go to bed each night knowing that if you died in your sleep you would leave the world a better place? Are your family relationships exceptional? Have you been a great friend? Is your financial house in order? Are systems and procedures at work in place so that if you were hit by a bus the business wouldn't fall apart? If the answers to these questions cause some anxiety, the feedback is to address these each and every day until you can fall asleep comfortably knowing that your life is exceptional on every level.

> *"We're going to shift from a win at all costs mentality to a win on all levels understanding."*
> *– Trevor Hendy*

What if you knew you only had 180 days to live?

If it all seems a bit too confronting that you could die in the next 24 hours – and you are yet to have your affairs in order – consider playing the 'game' that you will die in 180 days. Whilst highly unlikely, it's quite possible for any single one of us to die within the next six months.

If it weren't for this 180 Days to Live exercise you wouldn't be reading this book. Some years ago I ran this exercise in a small group workshop and decided to do it myself with the participants. After the group set some big life goals, I asked, "How would your goals change if you *knew* you were going to die in 180 days?" Instead of setting goals on business revenue and body fat percentage, people's responses included: "Organise my life insurance policy"; "spend more quality time with my partner and children"; "go on the holiday I keep putting off"; "read the book I've never made time for" and "play the piano I've been 'too busy' to enjoy".

For me, I decided that if I had 180 days to live I would want my children to have a manuscript from me on 'how to live'. There was no pressure for it to be published. Given my own love affair with books, I simply wanted my philosophy on life organised into words. Having run events, delivered speeches, hosted podcasts, written blogs and published online learning courses, I felt my message was too fractured for my children to know what I really thought about the art of living. I wanted a timeless manuscript that they could pick up at any stage of their life – from teenage years and onwards – and know that this is what I thought about life and how to live it.

I began getting up at 5am each morning, made myself a green tea and began typing out my key messages and thoughts in the eight key areas of life. Within 180 days, I had my manuscript, which became the first draft of the book you're reading now. That process began back in 2016, and so, whilst I didn't die in 180 days (thankfully), the knowledge that it was certainly possible drove me to get this book underway.

Exceptional Exercise 8.2: 180 Days To Live

Choose up to three important, non-urgent goals or actions you would want to take if you knew you would be dead in six months. Commit to achieve one of them. For some people, organising or updating a life insurance policy is the most important next step. For others, it's healing a family relationship. Looking your mortality in the eyes will not only bring a piercing clarity and incredible urgency to your life, it will massively reduce your fear of death, and provide you with a gratitude for your birth and life that allows you to be more fully present.

Conflict of Opposites 5: War and peace

World peace has often been the symbol for human perfection. Dozens of theories exist on how world peace could be achieved – communism, democracy and capitalism being just a few. Whilst war is a senseless and gross waste of human life, as long as there is peace we will always have war. Just as darkness allows us to define light, war allows us to define peace.

When I mention the words 'war' and 'peace' it's easy to think first of world wars and world peace. War, however, doesn't only happen on a world and civil scale. Whilst war tears countries apart, household warfare tears families and individuals apart. We might call it domestic violence, but let there be no mistaking: domestic violence feels like war to all involved. The notion that world peace can be achieved by removing world war doesn't address the potentially worse ramifications of household warfare.

> **Global household warfare**
> - The WHO estimates more than one in three women on the planet (35%) have experienced physical and/or sexual intimate partner violence or non-partner sexual violence in their lifetime. Globally, up to 38% of murdered women were killed by their male intimate partner.
> - More than 10 million Americans experience domestic violence each year
> - In Australia one domestic violence incidence takes place every two minutes. One in three women have experienced physical or sexual violence by someone known to them. Sexual assault and domestic violence are the most common crimes committed in Australia.

Source: World Health Organization [10]

There is no peace without war

As I write this, it's highly likely you live a relatively war-free peaceful life, but that doesn't mean war isn't a part of your existence. If you have children you probably experience 'war' of some kind on a daily or weekly basis, 'choosing your battles' about when to 'confront' your children on their behaviour. At some point during the battle the peacekeepers arrive by way of the other parent or another sibling. A truce is eventually called and a ceasefire takes place until the next inevitable battle. The same happens on the sporting field, in politics and in the workplace, where opposing departments, major competitors or disgruntled clients regularly wage a war of varying size in order to get what they want.

Yes, war has taught us many valuable principles on how to live. At its foundation, the brutality of war gives us great perspective on the beauty and preciousness of life. The peace we experience provides an urgency to end war as soon as possible, so that we can return to peacetime. Knowing that we are caught in the middle of both and will be for our entire life provides us with the opportunity to exercise compassion during 'war' times, gratitude during 'peace' times, and presence and love whilst stuck in the middle.

Conflict of Opposites 6: Poverty and wealth

More than 3.4 billion people live on less than US $5.50 per day.[11] All countries experience relative poverty, which can be calculated by finding the median income in your country and halving it. This amount is known as the poverty line or threshold. One in eight Australians, one in seven Americans and one in five UK citizens live in poverty, whilst 10% of the world live in *extreme* poverty (less than US $1.90 per day).[12]

Poverty is not solely based on income. Multidimensional poverty is a combination of causes and effects – poor health, lack of education, inadequate living standards, the threat of violence, unemployment or poor quality of work, environmental hazards and more, all contribute to a more rounded definition of poverty. For example, the poorest 40% of Australians are 71% more likely to commit suicide, obesity is 35%

more prevalent, activity levels are 22% lower and smoking rates are almost double.[13]

Whilst it's easy to blame the extremely wealthy for not eliminating 'poverty' (the richest 1% own 44% of the planet's wealth), multidimensional poverty shows us that it's unwise to think that money is the sole cure. Viewed more holistically, poverty provides a far greater opportunity than emptying the pockets of the rich. Helping others in dire need provides all of us – extremely wealthy or not – with a purpose to contribute beyond ourselves.

Poverty provides purpose

Whilst I've already outlined that money gives you more to be good with, poverty provides us all with a humanitarian purpose that nothing else can. Mother Teresa is perhaps the archetypal example of this, her deeds contributing to her canonisation by the Catholic Church in 2016, honoured as Saint Teresa of Calcutta.

Born in Albania, Mother Teresa left home at 18 to join the Sisters of Loreto in Ireland with a view of becoming a missionary. A year later she moved to India, where she took her religious vows at age 20 and became a teacher and eventually principal at St Mary's School in Kolkata. In 1946, deeply moved by the poverty surrounding her, Mother Teresa experienced a calling she described as the "call within a call".

"I was to leave the convent and help the poor while living among them," she reflected. "It was an order. To fail would have been to break the faith." Beginning her missionary work in 1948, Mother Teresa dedicated the remainder of her life – another 49 years – to helping the sick and poor in India and abroad. The Vatican received billions of dollars in donations as vision of her work spread across the globe. Mother Teresa's life purpose and her incredible example would not have been possible without the existence of poverty.

You don't need to be Mother Teresa or set foot in India to witness the humanitarian power and purpose that poverty provides. In the 2020 Australian bushfire disaster, an estimated one billion animals and 451 humans lost their lives. More than 45 million acres were burned and almost 10,000 buildings destroyed.

The environmental and social impact on top of the instant multidimensional poverty that the bushfires created stirred an unprecedented amount of generosity amongst the global population. Whilst the likes of international celebrities Pink and Leonardo DiCaprio donated in excess of $500,000 each, more than half of the Australian population (53%) donated funds. From young children breaking their piggy banks to Australian businessman Andrew Forrest donating $70 million, human beings used their relative wealth to show their support, whilst many used their wealth of time to volunteer in various ways.

Let's not forget that poverty of any kind – be it acute or chronic – pulls on our heartstrings. Poverty and wealth are yet another reminder that we are caught in the middle of an often excruciating conflict of opposites. So whilst it's noble and even inspiring to dedicate time and money to the relief and possible eradication of poverty, it's important to recognise that the very existence of the problem is what gives many of us the purpose, gratitude and compassion we need to live our exceptional life.

"All you see in the world is the outcome of your idea about it."
– Neale Donald Walsch

● ● ●

Lesson 3: The Spirit Has No Limits

So far in this chapter we've observed that pain in life is inevitable and that our life exists in a world filled with opposites. These first two steps are somewhat limiting, given that pain will have an end and that there are benefits to both sides of human experience.

When you can move beyond pain and the conflict of opposites, what remains is the soul. And your soul is limitless. Your soul doesn't have labels for good or bad, right or wrong, truth or lies. Some call the limitless soul pure love, consciousness or light. Some call it God, Allah, Buddha, Gaia, Pachamama or simply Universe. Whatever you call it, the soul renders its most aware students speechless, perhaps best exemplified by meditation, breath and sleep.

"Words reduce reality to something the human mind can grasp, which isn't very much," according to Eckhart Tolle. "Language consists of five basic sounds produced by the vocal cords. They are the vowels a, e, i, o, u. The other sounds are consonants produced by air pressure: s, f, g, and so forth. Do you believe some combination of such basic sounds could ever explain who you are, or the ultimate purpose of the universe, or even what a tree or stone is in its depth?"[14]

Spirit Limiter 1: Expectations

Earlier I mentioned Shakespeare's line: "Oft expectation fails, and most oft there where most it promises." Not just exclusive to relationships, expectations weigh heavily on the spirit. The height of mindfulness – in fact, fulfilment in life – is to remove most of the expectations you have on yourself, others and events. Expectations make life a game that's difficult to win and easy to lose, and their subsequent removal or reduction will greatly impact your spiritual fulfilment.

From sunny or rainy days, heavy or light traffic, tears of sorrow or tears of joy, your expectations are a spiritual invitation to take a bird's eye view on life and get some perspective. "Be the silent watcher of your thoughts and behaviour," said Tolle. "Rather than *being* your thoughts and emotions, be the awareness behind them. You are beneath the thinker. You are the stillness beneath the mental noise. You are the love and joy beneath the pain."[15]

The ABCDs of negativity

With that in mind, turn your attention to your specific expectations. There are at least 15 types of expectations you have on yourself, others, circumstances and inanimate objects such as your car, computer and phone. These unmet expectations cause us to feel what Dr John Demartini terms the *ABCDs of Negativity* –

A = Anger and aggression
B = Blame or betrayal
C = Criticism and challenge
D = Despair, depression or despondent[16]

Firstly, ask yourself which of these emotions you feel the most under stress or when expectations aren't met. When things seem to go against you are you likely to feel depressed, down or despondent? Perhaps you get angry and aggressive? Or you become intensely critical of yourself or others? Do you feel betrayed or play the blame game? I am most likely to be critical of myself or others. When I find myself being critical I realise I have had high expectations on myself or others that haven't been met.

According to Dr Demartini, expectations include –
- An unrealistic expectation on other people to be more like you (to have your values, do things your way or agree with you).
- An unrealistic expectation on others to be unlike themselves (for example, if I expected Sarah to love football – to be unlike herself and more like me).
- An unrealistic expectation on machines to work all the time (the car or phone battery runs flat, the computer freezes or Wi-Fi is slow).
- An unrealistic expectation on yourself or others to be one-sided (to be happy *all* the time).
- An unrealistic expectation on God or higher power to live outside universal laws and/or inside your values (reach your goals every time on time, the sun to shine every day of your holiday, only the elderly to die and not the young).[17]

To reiterate, unrealistic expectations will cause you heartache. If you currently have heartache in your life – whether directed towards yourself, family, friends, colleagues, politicians, a higher power or inanimate objects – it is purely because your expectation hasn't been met. Many times, you don't know that you have the expectation until you feel the heartache. That's why being aware of your expectations can be so powerful. When you realise that it's *you* that is creating the stress for yourself (because of your expectation), it's relatively easy to identify the cause of your stress. Then it's time to do something about it (as outlined in the section on family).

Spirit Limiter 2: Fear

"Fear defeats more people than any other thing in the world," wrote American philosopher Ralph Waldo Emerson. What stops many from living an exceptional life is not opportunity or genes or status, it's the fearful and often false thoughts we allow into our mind. It could be the fear to go against the advice of family, the fear to leave the secure job or the fear to ask someone on a date. No matter the fear, it is entirely our creation and no one else's.

We fear something not because of fear itself, but because we fear rejection if our greatest fears come true. To feel rejected is to fear the loss of being loved or liked, and for many people to feel unloved is to feel worthless. And to feel worthless brings with it an attitude of not giving 100% to life. This domination of fear on our life is what the Dalai Lama has acknowledged surprises him the most about human beings. "He is so anxious about the future that he does not enjoy the present," he says. "The result being that he does not live in the present or the future; he lives as if he is never going to die, and then dies having never really lived."

There are numerous ways to interpret the Dalai Lama's comments. It's easy to visualise 'never going to die' as a reckless, 'invincible' party-loving person (particularly if you're under 30). Instead, this statement refers to taking the easy way out and staying in the job you hate, holding on to the toxic relationship for fear of loneliness, or eating junk food like it's wholefood. If we lived with a spiritual urgency that our days in this life are numbered (which they are), we would make the hard calls more courageously. If we lived our life really knowing the clock is ticking, we might prioritise our exceptional life over the easier, less exceptional one. Instead, many of us strain our way through life and get to our final breath 'having never really lived'.

The antidote to fear is courage

To turn life around requires living with the opposite of fear, and that is courage. To live with fear is to live according to the expectations of others, whilst to live with courage is to live life on your own terms. It's not easy and it's not always fun, but courage builds a spiritual muscle that conquers fear. It often requires doing things in spite of fear, and the more fear you have when you do something, the more courageous your behaviour is often perceived to be.

"It's not the mountain we conquer, but ourselves," reflected Sir Edmund Hillary, the first human to scale the summit of Mount Everest (alongside Tenzing Norgay) in 1953. We all have metaphorical mountains in our lives – seemingly insurmountable tasks or barriers in work, family, health and wealth – but it's not the barriers that are the problem; it's our attitude about the barriers and resultant fear or courage that determines the outcome.

> *"Don't ever fear to fail. Be inspired to succeed."*
> *– Sam Saggers*

Fear is your friend

In this way, fear is your friend, not your foe. It can be the signpost or guide in times of danger and trouble. But when your basic needs – food, water, warmth, rest, security and safety – are met, fear is just another speed bump to drive over in life. Some will do it by speeding up, some will slowly crawl over it. Either way, however you choose to 'get over it', your exceptional life is waiting for you on the other side.

Yes, there will be fear in place whilst you kill the fear, and that's where you can only surrender and do as Susan Jeffers proclaimed in her book with the same name: "Feel the fear and do it anyway." There exists an incredible mistruth in popular culture that you can and should be fearless. It's a complete myth. If anything makes you fearless, it is practice. And even still, if you are fearless, you risk becoming complacent, which opens you up to mistakes, which is then likely to lower your confidence and create anxiety and increase your fear. So, embrace your fear. Beware of fear generated by the media or perpetuated by your family and friends, but welcome the fear that challenges you to be exceptional.

> *"Today is the tomorrow you worried about yesterday."*
> *– Dale Carnegie*

Spirit Limiter 3: Judgement

"Love is the absence of judgement," according to the Dalai Lama, whilst Mother Teresa said it this way: "If you judge people, you have no time to love them." If you reflect for a moment and ask yourself how unconditionally you love and how loved you feel, you'll get an insight as to how much judgement exists in your life.

When judgement is low and love is high, it is far easier to accept other human beings for who they are. The exceptional life of Holocaust survivor Celina Biniaz was arguably kick-started by the non-judgement of a semi-cloistered nun, Mother Leontina. Not having access to the news of the world, the elderly nun taught Biniaz English and German without any prejudice towards Jews.

"She was the first human being who accepted me for who I was – a 14-year-old girl who needed help," recalls Biniaz, who was tutored by Mother Leontina shortly after the liberation. Her mentor's non-judgement was contagious, infecting Biniaz and helping her reflect on her traumatic experiences with grace. "I learned that you can never walk in another person's shoes," Biniaz told me on *100 Not Out*. "You can never predict how you would act in any situation. I've become much less judgemental on other people's actions because you never know what motivated that person to do what they did."

The shortcut to reducing judgement in your life is to become intensely curious. "We have two ears and one mouth so that we can listen twice as much as we speak," proclaimed Greek philosopher Epictetus. Our judgements are almost always made in statements and talking, whilst our curiosity is reflected with questions and listening.

Judgemental Statements	Curious questions
I hate my job.	What is my dissatisfaction at work telling me?
I hate my body.	What is the opportunity my body is presenting me with right now?
Today has been a great day.	What have been the challenges in the day to be wary of?
I'll be happy when I'm rich.	How can I be happy *whilst* I endeavour to grow my wealth?

Testing your limitless soul

If you truly believe the soul is limitless, you will find the limits being tested every day. If you believe that everything happens for a reason and a purpose that serves your exceptional life, events will happen in your life that truly *test* this belief. Family challenges, business challenges, health crises and so on will constantly be testing your belief in the grace and perfection of life.

If you choose to test the limits of your spirit, you are consciously deciding to live an exceptional life. In fact, whatever age you are now is the best time to open your soul up to the magnificence of the world.

Wherever you are now in life, start here. But know that if you choose this path it's not going to be easy; it will be the biggest and most powerful decision you can ever make in your life.

When you take control and consciously write the script of your own life, you are removing the addictions of being the victim, of labelling everything and everyone, and you no longer have an alibi or excuse for settling for average. Unleashing your limitless soul is not easy, but it is the most important work you'll ever do.

▲ ▲ ▲

Lesson 4: Not All Spiritual Practices are Created Equal

As you go about living your exceptional life you will undoubtedly dabble or immerse yourself in a spiritual practice of some kind. It is arguable that we have forgotten what the art of spiritual *practice* really is. If you take a look at the Ladder of Spiritual Practice, you'll see six activities – sleep, breath, prayer, gratitude, meditation and mindfulness. All of them have their own workshops, seminars, hashtags, apps and cult followings. Sleep and breath are arguably the two most important nutrients to sustaining human life. Sadly, both are often neglected in the conversation of spiritual health, shunted to the more tangible physical realm. Many children naturally sink in to the six spiritual practices quite effortlessly (watching newborn babies sleep and breathe is magic). Yet as we get older, we seemingly forget how to do one or all of these six activities well, and we therefore need to relearn them by unlearning some of our poor habits that have created a less than perfect environment for our exceptional spirit.

Mastering all six at once is not essential in order to thrive spiritually. Over time, as you consciously create your exceptional life, you will naturally embody all six practices. For now, this section is your invitation to reclaim and improve at least one of the practices that you know will allow you to take the next big step forward in your life.

> *"Spiritual practice is not just sitting and meditation. Practice is looking, thinking, touching, drinking, eating and talking. Every act, every breath, and every step can be practice and can help us to become more ourselves."*
> — ***Thich Nhat Hanh***

The Ladder of Spiritual Practice

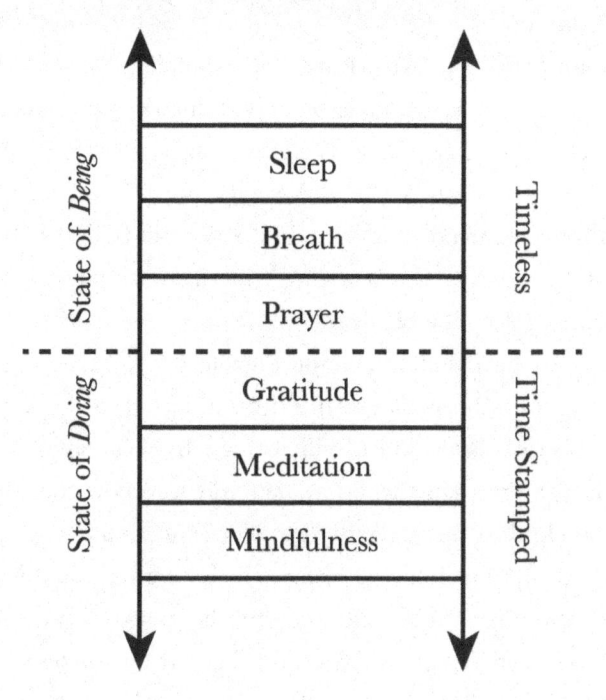

	State of *Being*		
	Sleep		Timeless
	Breath		
	Prayer		
---	---	---	---
	Gratitude		Time Stamped
State of *Doing*	Meditation		
	Mindfulness		

Spiritual Practice 1: Sleep

"Sleep is the best meditation," according to the Dalai Lama and the Cleveland Clinic's Dr Michael Roizen calls it "the most underrated health habit". Either we're beginning to lose trust in sage advice or too many people simply aren't aware of the power of sleep.

I'm often asked where sleep fits in to the Exceptional Life Blueprint. There's no doubt in my mind that sleep is as important for our spiritual health as it is for our physical, mental and emotional wellbeing.

Like most parents, my relationship with sleep intensified when my daughter, Maya, was born in 2010. Before then, I completely overrated sleep. I subscribed to Arnold Schwarzenegger's heroic mantra of "sleep faster". And while Schwarzenegger sleeps six hours per night (so that he can do more of what he loves in the remaining 18), most people's poor sleep quality and quantity is due to lifestyle choices and poor working environments.

More than a third of Americans, for example, sleep less than seven hours per night, with the average at 6.8 hours. Approximately 20% have a sleep disorder, and since 1985 the number of people sleeping *less* than six hours has risen by 31%. A staggering 97% of teenagers sleep less than the recommended amount, and seven out of every 10 university students sleep poorly. Costing the American taxpayers more than US $400 billion, sleep is a big deal.[18]

So why do we have such little respect for sleep?

When a child is born, one of the first things they do is go to sleep (no doubt entering the world is exhausting)! In their days as an infant, they're asleep more than they're awake, and we know that this sleep is vital for the child to thrive. As we get older we need less sleep than we did as a child. But our body's systems – including our nervous, immune, endocrine, and digestive – still require the parasympathetic nervous system to 'rest and repair' or 'rest and digest'. This takes a significant amount of time, which many of us are not giving to ourselves. Sleep performs a countless number of tasks, from slowing our heart rate, increasing immune activity, growing muscle, repairing tissue and synthesising hormones.

Emotionally, it's much easier to be happy after a good night's sleep. Mentally, it's far easier to concentrate and solve problems after a solid sleep. And spiritually, when you consider the conflict of opposites, the judgement, expectations and other challenges we face daily, we are far more tolerant and accepting of these after a good sleep.

When you add an exceptional morning ritual to a good night's sleep, you can reap incredible rewards. If you're resistant to any of this, simply go a night without sleep and compare your mental, emotional and spiritual performance to that of a day when you have a good night's sleep. When you give yourself the gift of an exceptional sleep on a daily basis, just like compound interest, your physical, mental and emotional health can improve exponentially.

Importantly, if you are in the midst of significant challenge, going to bed grateful for your problems is vital (problems are a sign of life, after all). If you do work you love you will end the day inspired and mentally fatigued (that's a good thing). If you move regularly you will sleep better, because your body will naturally want the rest. If you socialise throughout the day you will more happily enjoy time to yourself at bedtime hours. If you nourish your body and avoid stimulants at night you will improve your chances of a good night's rest. If you show or tell your family members each night before bed how much you love them, you'll sleep well.

If your evening ritual includes reading a book at night (with a lamp on, not a full blown downlight) you are likely to fall asleep more easily (unless it's a thriller). Avoid the temptation to stare at a screen for hours or browse social media. Neither will give you a good night's sleep. If you've been wise with your money during the day you will fall asleep more easily. If you are thankful for your life and communicate this through prayer, meditation, journaling or contemplation, you will be more at ease when you go to bed.

Morning and evening rituals

Whilst there still exists a great divide in the philosophy of sleep and the recommended hours each of us gets, what everyone agrees on is the importance of a ritual or rhythm to begin and end each day.

Each morning when I wake I simply want to get moving. I've gone through periods of my life where I've risen at 4am, meditated for thirty minutes, followed by yoga, a run, a green juice while writing in my gratitude journal before enjoying a nutrient-dense breakfast. After a few months my morning routine was exhausting. Now, all I feel the urge to do to start my day off exceptionally is to move my body. It typically lasts anywhere between 20 minutes and an hour. I belive it's important to find your 'one thing' for an exceptional morning so that you aren't relying on *everything* going your way in order to start the day well.

My evening ritual includes anything that doesn't involve a screen. It often consists of reconnecting with Sarah and learning. If Sarah hasn't gone to bed early, we'll sit down with a cup of herbal tea and chat about the day. Sarah goes to bed no later than 9pm most weekdays and I tend to stay up for an hour or so after, reading a book. On the weekends I break all my weekday rituals and replace the book for a movie on the couch with Sarah.

> **Poor sleep's brutal wake up call**
> Arianna Huffington, founder of *The Huffington Post* and author of *The Sleep Revolution*, collapsed from exhaustion at her desk in 2007. She woke up in a pool of blood with a fractured cheekbone. Her 18-hour days having caught up with her, she changed her entire life to pay sleep the respect it deserved. Huffington founded Thrive Global, a company dedicated to supporting individuals struggling with stress and burnout.

Spiritual Practice 2: Breath

In July of 1995, on the first day of the *Running of the Bulls* in Pamplona, Spain, Wim Hof's (b. 1959) life was about to change forever. Hof was a 35-year old husband and father of four when his wife jumped off her parent's eighth story apartment balcony, ending her life. After a long battle with schizophrenia, Olaya Hof's death was the catalyst for her husband's life purpose.

"She was the love of my life," Hof recounted in an episode of *The Rich Roll Podcast*.[19] "Grief is something very abstract. Whatever is inside you can't console it. You have to go deep. I began to look into nature. I found relief of a broken heart in the freezing water. Your mind shuts down and is just there, breaking the loop of possible emotional deep grief. My kids made me survive; nature healed me."[20]

Combining cold exposure, breathwork and meditation (which Hof calls "commitment"), Hof began to renew his life and simultaneously garner the attention of the world's research community. His practice, known as the Wim Hof Method, has been shown to reduce stress, chronic pain and inflammation, improve sleep, recovery, creativity, focus and mental clarity.

Hof is the holder of 26 Guinness World Records including the fastest barefoot half marathon on snow. He reached the 'death zone' of Everest – an altitude of 7,200 metres – in nothing but shorts and ice boots. At the time of print his world-record ice bath duration sits at 1 hour, 52 minutes and 42 seconds.

Generally speaking, human beings can go roughly three weeks without food, three days without water and three minutes without oxygen. Whilst Hof can hold his breath for 10 minutes, the point is that oxygen is more important than water, which is more important than food. Sadly, society gets this inversely twisted. We tend to overeat, are chronically dehydrated and pay little attention to breathing properly. Many of us still believe that breathing has no impact on our level of health.

Breathing practices have been part of many cultures for centuries, and hundreds exist today. In Indigenous Australian culture, circular breathing is used to master playing the didgeridoo. Whether it's pranayama, Buteyko breathing or the Wim Hof Method – all practices have their place. Some focus on deep diaphragmatic breathing, pursed lips or alternate nostril breathing. Your job is to breathe in a way that supports your exceptional life. You don't need to be like Wim Hof and learn how to hold your breath for 10 minutes. Instead it's vital to recognise when shallow breathing appears (often under stress). It's important to develop the art of deep breathing and use it as a lifestyle, a stress reduction technique and opportunity to connect with your limitless spirit.

Spiritual Practice 3: Prayer

When faith is low, desperation can be high and the reverse is also true. Prayer arguably builds the spiritual muscles of faith, trust and certainty unlike any other practice. One could argue that those who pray most regularly have the strongest spiritual muscle – including the evangelists and the zealots. They have a certainty – a conviction – that we may not agree with, but its strength has been largely built on prayer and an extreme devotion.

The more you pray, chant, or affirm your wishes and gratitude for your exceptional life (and the lives of others), the more you give yourself the opportunity to build an unshakable faith, trust and conviction that you are exactly where you need to be and that the rest of your life will be the best of your life. Hoping and wishing for an exceptional life does not give you that conviction. In fact, hoping for things to change is only the first step. Hope plus intention plus prayer plus regular action plus reviewing or reflecting upon your results is the cycle which *The Exceptionals* naturally follow.

Prayer is not only for the religious

In a poll of more than 2000 UK residents conducted by Christian aid agency, Tearfund, 51% of them acknowledged that they pray.[21]

Just under half of those who pray said they believed their God or higher power hears their prayers. Four in 10 felt that prayer changes the world with a similar number saying it makes them feel better. Family is the most common prayer subject (71%), followed by thanking God (42%), praying for healing (40%), friends (40%) and poverty or global disaster (24%).[22]

Interestingly, one in five agnostics said that they prayed, with personal crisis or tragedy the most common reason for doing so. One of the respondents was 64-year-old Henry, who when asked if he believed in God, said: "I don't know but I would describe myself at the sceptical end of agnosticism. I certainly wouldn't classify myself as religious." Yet Henry prays every night, kneeling by his bed, beginning with a silent recitation of the Lord's Prayer followed by prayers for his loved ones to be kept safe and well.[23]

"Sometimes I include other specific people or suffering groups," says Henry. "Then I have a fuzzy moment about me – not concrete thoughts, and I don't ask for specific things." Asked about his somewhat ritualised praying, Henry said: "I worry about it quite a lot – is it some kind of an insurance policy, is it superstition or is it something more real?"[24]

Whatever the case for Henry or yourself, prayer is an avenue to bring about more faith, trust and certainty, but not necessarily material gifts. "Prayer can involve requests, but it's unhelpful to see God as a heavenly Santa," says Isabelle Hamley, chaplain to the Archbishop of Canterbury. "Prayer is primarily a line of communication with God – thinking, reflecting, bringing one's concerns and worries into a bigger picture."[25]

If you're not religious, and you're on the 'sceptical side of agnosticism' like Henry, just do as Henry does and pray anyway – even if you have no idea who you're praying to. You really do have nothing to lose except for the time it takes, and the best place to start is with gratitude.

> *"My heart is at ease knowing that what*
> *was meant for me will never miss me.*
> *And what misses me was never meant for me."*
> *– Sufi prayer*

Spiritual Practice 4: Gratitude

As mentioned, gratitude is one of the most common themes of prayer. Being grateful is encouraged in many religions as a noble character trait and has been a key pillar of philosophy since ancient times. At the turn of the 21st century, gratitude had risen in popular culture to such an extent that it became the subject of much study as to its emotional and therapeutic benefits.

Society has been subsequently inundated with books, journals, techniques and reasons for having a gratitude practice. As a result, gratitude has found its way on the to-do list for many people's morning and evening rituals. The accomplishment of being grateful for a few minutes each day gets ticked off the list, with the endorphin rush of achieving gratitude titillating the grateful individual for a fleeting moment or two. In my opinion, that's not what gratitude is about.

For *The Exceptionals*, gratitude is a way of being *and* doing. It's an innate, somewhat unconscious way to live. The graceful agers that I have met and interviewed have grateful personalities. It comes across as an optimism and sense of joy or fulfilment – an 'attitude of gratitude' (as cliché as it sounds) – in even the simplest pleasures: the smile of a young child, the sun shining, the apple ripening on the tree or the love from a warm embrace. Whilst most *Exceptionals* I know survive without a gratitude journal, they do have a faith in a higher power that sees them praying regularly and giving thanks. In other words, you can experience incredible gratitude without a gratitude journal. Before gratitude journals existed or were conceived, there was prayer, speech, meditation and reflective thoughts. The art of exceptional gratitude is an authentic combination of *being* grateful and *doing* gratitude. What's important is finding the unique blend that works for you.

Exceptional Exercise 8.3: How grateful are you?

If you want to do your own research study, take a test to find out how grateful you are now and then take the same test one week, then one month, and then three months later. There are many tests that help you define your state of gratitude at present. Three of the most referenced are the GQ6 test, the GRAT assessment and Appreciation Scale. They are all quick and easy to complete. Links to each one are available at **marcuspearce.com.au/yourexceptionallife**

> *"Let gratitude be the pillow upon which you kneel to say your nightly prayer. And let faith be the bridge you build to overcome evil and welcome good."*
> *– Maya Angelou*

Spiritual Practice 5: Meditation

Just like many people are attempting to do gratitude without being grateful, modern society has been inundated with techniques, books and courses on how to do meditation without so much as a reference to being meditative. For those looking for the silver bullet to an exceptional spirit, simply 'doing' meditation won't make you more spiritual.

The intense focus on doing meditation has left many frustrated and hating on themselves for not being able to meditate, when in fact nothing could be further from the truth. Coupled with the culturally driven propaganda that we should all have a meditation practice in order to sustain our mental health and happiness, meditation – and being able to do it successfully – has descended into a form of status symbol and measure of enlightenment.

Hundreds of meditation practices exist today and there is no one clear definition of meditation. Some recommend focusing on one thing (or one mantra) whilst others suggest reaching a point of no thoughts and finding 'the gap' in between thoughts. From mantra-based meditation (such as Transcendental Meditation), breathwork, Zen, Clear Light, Golden Light and a litany of guided meditations, it's easy to see why people get confused and overwhelmed and feel apprehensive upon beginning a meditation practice.

But what if there was a way to successfully meditate that doesn't feel as unattainable as many make it out to be? And what if you already did it without knowing?

How to live meditatively

In 2019 I was interviewed for a documentary called *The Longevity Film*. Filmmaker Kale Brock travelled to the Japanese island of Okinawa, the Greek island of Ikaria and the Californian city of Loma Linda – three of the world's Blue Zones – in order to discover the reasons for their exceptional quantity and quality of life.

Up until travelling to shoot the film, Brock had a regular Transcendental Meditation (TM) practice that lasted 20 minutes in the morning and night. "I had done a course and I had been dabbling in meditation when it was appropriate. Everyone had been talking about TM and I had heard about how good it was, so I felt like I had to do it," Brock told me. "I felt like if I didn't do it I was missing out on something."

Whilst in Ikaria, Brock was helping local farmer Ilias Parikos pick strawberries when he had what he described as a "peak moment" of insight. "The final straw was watching Ilias and how hard he was working in the garden. The way he did it was just so calm and graceful and present, especially given these were regular, seemingly inane activities. The work seemed to have this great effect on him – he was so happy and relaxed. I was like 'why in the modern world are we trying to shortcut to *that* moment when we have all of these opportunities available to us in how we live every day? We don't need to meditate to get there. We just need to live more meditatively.'"

There is a Zen proverb that states: "Before enlightenment, chop wood, carry water. After enlightenment, chop wood, carry water." Similarly, my view is: "Before meditating, see the extraordinary in the ordinary. After meditating, see the extraordinary in the ordinary." By all means, have a meditation practice if you are inclined to. And when you're not meditating, live meditatively.

Spiritual Practice 6: Mindfulness

The concept of mindfulness is a relatively modern term in popular culture, however the practice of it is as old as Buddhism itself. There seem to be many definitions for mindfulness, all boiling down to mastering the art of being fully present in the moment. Mindfulness practices may include meditation, breathing, yoga, journaling, colouring, painting, listening, walking, active listening, spending time in nature and more. In the context of this book, mindfulness is a combination of meditative activities, including meditation itself.

▲ ▲ ▲

Don't Overbake the Spirit Cake

I know too many people who breathe well, meditate like a champion, and won't forgive their spouse for having an affair. I know devout Catholics who pray religiously, yet eat too much and never exercise and complain about poor sleep. Be mindful of overbaking the spirit cake whilst settling for mediocrity in the other key areas of life.

At the same time, when inevitable stress and pain occurs, relying on spiritual practices is far more effective than over the counter medications, junk food, alcohol and other quick-fix remedies. By focusing on a spiritual practice like getting a good night's sleep, you'll inevitably find your ability to deal with stress far greater. If that feels easier said than done, you might choose to focus on breath, prayer, gratitude, meditation and mindfulness. Choose these practices first before you resort to the quick fixes. And if you still find your stress levels difficult to manage, be sure to identify which area of your exceptional life is causing you stress, and ensure you are applying the principles outlined in the relevant section.

The drowning devotee on the rooftop

You may have heard the following story of the wishful thinker sitting on a roof:

> A fellow was stuck on his rooftop in a flood.
> He was praying to God for help.
> Soon a man in a rowboat came by and
> the fellow shouted to the man on the roof,
> "Jump in, I can save you."
>
> The stranded fellow shouted back,
> "No, it's OK, I'm praying to God and
> He is going to save me."
>
> So the rowboat went on.

Then a motorboat came by.
The fellow in the motorboat shouted,
"Jump in, I can save you."

To this the stranded man said,
"No thanks, I'm praying to God and
He is going to save me. I have faith."

So the motorboat went on.

Then a helicopter came by and
the pilot shouted down,
"Grab this rope and I will lift you to safety."

To this the stranded man again replied,
"No thanks, I'm praying to God and
He is going to save me. I have faith."

So the helicopter reluctantly flew away.

Soon the water rose above the rooftop and
the man drowned. He went to Heaven.
He finally got his chance to discuss this
whole situation with God,
at which point he exclaimed,
"I had faith in you but you didn't save me,
you let me drown. I don't understand why!"

To this God replied,
"I sent you a rowboat and a motorboat and
a helicopter, what more did you expect?"

As you go about crafting your exceptional life, you'll find yourself sitting on the rooftop many times. Your challenge is to observe the rowboat, the motorboat and the helicopter and gratefully accept support when it is offered. See the miracle in every day and in every person you come into contact with. Remember that *Your Exceptional Life* is a script written by two authors – you and some form of higher power. Never forget your role and responsibility in writing it. You must write first. Show whatever higher power you believe in that you have the courage to take responsibility for the incredible gift you have been given – your life – and go about it with a grace and reverence that brings about everyday miracles rather than spending precious time on the rollercoaster of enlightenment or the ever-yearning futile search for the one day when the world will be enlightened en masse.

Now is the time to go ahead and put your spirit into everything, without any limits whatsoever. Put your heart and soul into the work you do, the way you care for your body, the friendships you create in your life, the family you were born into and raise, the knowledge you accumulate and apply in your life, the financial wealth you generate, and of course your relationship with yourself and the planet.

Give yourself the gift of living with a limitless soul and watch the rest of your life truly become the *best* of your life.

AFTERWORD

If you're overwhelmed right now at the task of living your exceptional life, then a part of me feels I've done my job and the other part feels compassion for you! Such is the bigness and brutality of life that recognising that you can and deserve to live your exceptional life is a titanic realisation. With that, some overwhelm at the size of the task ahead is only natural.

I encourage you to complete the Exceptional Exercises and download the adjoining workbook if you haven't already. Go to **marcuspearce.com.au/yourexceptionallife** to access the full set of resources. Much of what was cut from the 120,000 word manuscript is also located on this website, including profiles of many *Exceptionals* and an ebook called *Too Exceptional: The Inconvenient Truth of Mastering One Area of Life at the Expense of Others*.

Whether you apply a little or a lot from this book, my big hope for you is that you truly believe you can make the rest of your life the best of your life. Your beliefs determine your actions, and only you are in charge of your beliefs. People will die and challenges will crop up at the most unexpected times. Through all of this, your beliefs and philosophies will be what gets you through. My hope is that this book has taught you one of the most powerful beliefs you can have is to aim for exceptional in every area of life – not just one – as mastering one area of life at the expense of the others risks turmoil.

Thank you for giving my work and message so much of your precious time. May you continue to shine a light on living an exceptional life with your loved ones, and I one day hope to meet you in person and learn about your exceptional life.

Until then, make the rest of your life the best of your life.

All my love,
Marcus

ACKNOWLEDGEMENTS

Each time I read an author's acknowledgements I'm reminded how much of a team effort birthing a book is. I am no different in wanting to thank a number of exceptional souls who helped this book land in your hands.

Firstly to my children – Maya, Darby, Tommy and Spencer – you were the reason I decided to turn my thoughts and research into a book. I never believed I had a book inside me until you began arriving in the world.

Countless early mornings and weekends were spent writing this book at the expense of quality family time or helping around the house. To my angel sent from heaven, my incredible wife, Sarah. Your love, support and encouragement of me and the message I share has no limits. I am eternally grateful to you Bubsy.

To my brother from another mother, Damian Kristof. Your fingerprints are all over this book. If you never agreed to co-host *100 Not Out*, who knows what would have happened? The guests we have interviewed, the people whose lives our podcast and events have impacted and the experiences we have enjoyed together have all stemmed from your willingness to come on board.

Thank you to *The Exceptionals*. I owe a great deal to every single one of you. Without you this book would be paper-thin! I owe a special thank you to *The Exceptionals* who gave up their time to be interviewed on *100 Not Out* – Eddie Jaku, Dexter Kruger, Madonna Buder, Ruth Frith, Sanduk Ruit, Bronnie Ware, Cyndi O'Meara, Normie Rowe, Thelma Zimmerman, Jan Smith, John Demartini, Don Riddington, Heather Lee, Walter Bortz, Charles Eugster, Thea Parikos, Ruth Heidrich, Mimi Kirk, Bill Stevens, Trevor Hendy, Marc Cohen, Ada Murkies, Celina Biniaz, Kim Morrison and Kale Brock. To *The Exceptionals* who I couldn't squeeze into the final manuscript, thank you for your incredible influence in shaping my message.

To my professional mentors – among them Tony Robbins, Bob Proctor, Napoleon Hill, Brian Tracy, Jack Canfield, Wayne Dyer, John Robbins, Sir Ken Robinson, Robert Greene, Jason Whitton, Malcolm Gladwell and Victor Hugo – your life's work has influenced me greatly and provided me with multiple epiphanies, light-bulb moments and awakenings.

A special thank you to Dr John Demartini. Without your own dedication to your exceptional life purpose, I doubt that I would have found mine. Thank you for your support of this book and my message. I am eternally grateful.

To the wonderful people of Ikaria, particularly the village of Nas. Thea Parikos, if it wasn't for the love of yourself and your extended family, much of this book would have no foundation. Efharisto poli. And to Dan Buettner, author of *The Blue Zones*. If it wasn't for your book, I may never have found Ikaria.

To my teammates past and present at The Wellness Couch podcast network – namely Damian Kristof, Brett Hill, Laurence Tham, Kim Morrison, Cyndi O'Meara and Carren Smith. It has been an honour to go on such a wonderful adventure with you all.

To Candy Baker, your incredibly honest and thorough first edit was just what the book needed. To Natalie Deane, Jazmine Morales, Susan Dean and the team at Dean Publishing, thank you for helping me get to the finish line. Without you, this book would have been mediocre at best.

ACKNOWLEDGEMENTS

To the 40 people who first joined the *Exceptional Life Blueprint* program in 2014. Your decision to invest in my message was the confirmation I needed to commit my life to this work. I especially want to thank those members who read the manuscript, when it was gargantuan and overdetailed. A special thanks to Kate Raines, Peter Lennon and Laura Barry for your detailed feedback. To Bronnie Ware, Cyndi O'Meara and Kim Morrison who were very clear that my 120,000-word manuscript was closer to an encyclopedia than a regular book. And to Sam Gowing for your personal friendship and professional guidance from start to finish.

And finally to my immediate and wider family. Rob and Jill, you've raised an exceptional family which I am so thankful to be a part of. To Brenda, Josh, Leigh, Ashleigh, Penny, Chris and my extended family, thank you for who you are and the wonderful contribution you make to my life. To my sisters Olivia and Georgia, I love you both so much. I love that our love for each other grows the older we get.

To my beautiful Mother Darling – thank you for being you. You have taught me the power of personality, socialising, living for today, persistence, faith and fun. To DP, my best mate and incredible dad. The sacrifices you have made in your life for the betterment of others including myself inspires me every day to live my own exceptional life.

BIBLIOGRAPHY AND RECOMMENDED READING

If this book has inspired you, it's because so many books have inspired me to write this one. Hundreds of books were read and researched in order to write *Your Exceptional Life*. Here is a list of more than 60 works that have had a profound influence on the creation of this book.

Agassi, Andre (2009) *Open*, Alfred A Knopf, New York.

Albom, Mitch (1997) *Tuesdays with Morrie*. Doubleday, New York.

Bono, Tim (2018) *When Likes Aren't Enough*, Grand Central Life & Style, Hachette Book Group, New York.

Bortz, Walter M (2010) *The Roadmap To 100: The Breakthrough Science of Living a Long and Healthy Life*, St Martin's Press, New York.

Branson, Richard (2017) *Finding My Virginity*. Portfolio, Penguin Random House, New York.

Branson, Richard (2005) *Losing My Virginity*, revised edition, Random House Australia, New South Wales.

Buder, Madonna (2010). *The Grace to Race: The Wisdom and Inspiration of the 80-Year-Old World Champion Triathlete Known as the Iron Nun*, Simon & Schuster, New York.

Buettner, Dan (2010) *The Blue Zones: Lessons for Living Longer from the People Who Have Lived the Longest*, National Geographic Society, Washington.

Bruhn, John G. and Stewart Wolf (1979) *The Roseto Story: An Anatomy of Health*, University of Oklahoma Press, Oklahoma.

Carnegie, Dale (1998) *How To Win Friends and Influence People: The Only Book You Need to Lead You to Success*, revised edition, Pocket Books, Simon & Schuster, New York.

Chapman, Gary (1992) *The 5 Love Languages: How to Express Heartfelt Commitment to Your Mate*. Chicago, Northfield Publishing.

Clason, George S (2002) *The Richest Man in Babylon*, Signet, Penguin Group, United States.

Coelho, Paulo (1993) *The Alchemist*, HarperOne, HarperCollins Publishers, New York.

Covey, Stephen R (2004) *The 7 Habits of Highly Effective People: Powerful Lessons in Personal Change*, revised edition, Free Press, New York.

Daniher, Neale and Warwick Green (2019) *When All Is Said and Done*, Pan Macmillan Australia, Sydney.

Davis, William (2011) *Wheat Belly*, Rodale Books, United States.

Demartini, John (2004) *How to Make One Hell of a Profit and Still get to Heaven*, Hay House, United States.

Demartini, John (2002) *The Breakthrough Experience: A Revolutionary New Approach to Personal Transformation*, Hay House, United States.

Demartini, John (2013) *The Values Factor: The Secret to Creating an Inspired and Fulfilling Life*, The Berkley Publishing Group, Penguin Group, New York.

Dunn, Elizabeth and Edward Norton (2014) *Happy Money: The Science of Happier Spending*, Simon & Schuster, New York.

Eugster, Charles (2017) *Age is Just a Number: What a 97 Year Old Record Breaker Can Teach Us About Growing Older*, Sphere, Little, Brown Book Group, Hachette UK: London.

Favilli, Elena and Francesca Cavallo (2017) *Good Night Stories for Rebel Girls*, Particular Books, Penguin Random House, London.

Fiddian. Marc (1980) *Lines in the Anderson Tartan: The Harry Anderson story of sheer success*. Self-published, Australia.

Fonda, Jane (2011) *Prime Time: Love, Health, Sex, Fitness, Friendship, Spirit; Making the Most of all Your Life*, Random House, New York.

Frankl, Viktor (2006) *Man's Search For Meaning*, Beacon Press, Massachusetts.

Gibran, Kahlil (1923) *The Prophet*, Penguin Random House, New York.

Gladwell, Malcolm (2008) *Outliers*, Little, Brown and Company, Hachette Book Group, United States.

Grandin, Temple (2006) *Thinking in Pictures*, 2nd edition, Bloomsbury Publishing, London.

Greene, Robert (2012) *Mastery*, Profile Books, London.

Gripper, Ali (2018) *The Barefoot Surgeon: The Inspirational Story of Dr Sanduk Ruit, the Eye Surgeon Giving Sight and Hope to the World's Poor*, Allen & Unwin, Crows Nest, New South Wales.

Hill, Napoleon (2009) *Think and Grow Rich*, reproduced edition, Capstone Publishing, John Wiley & Sons, West Sussex.

Huffington, Arianna (2017) *The Sleep Revolution: Transforming Your Life, One Night at a Time*, Harmony Books, Crown Publishing Group, Penguin Random House, New York.

Isaacson, Walter (2008) *Einstein: His Life and Universe*, Simon & Schuster, New York.

Isaacson, Walter (2011) *Steve Jobs: The Exclusive Biography*, Simon & Schuster, New York.

Jaku, Eddie (2020) *The Happiest Man on Earth*, Pan Macmillan, Sydney.

Keller, Helen (1903) *The Story of My Life*, Doubleday, Page and Co, New York.

Kelly, Vikki (2016) *Mindful 2.0: An Ultimate Formula for Inner Bliss and a Meaningful Life*, Innate Wisdom.

Kiyosaki, Robert (2017) *Rich Dad Poor Dad*, 2nd edition, Plata Publishing, Scottsdale.

Kwik, Jim (2020) *Limitless*, Hay House, Carlsbad, California.

Mandela, Nelson (1994) *Long Walk to Freedom*, Little, Brown and Company, London.

Martinez, Mario (2014) *Mind Body Code: How to Change the Beliefs That Limit Your Health, Longevity, and Success*, Sounds True, Boulder, Colorado.

Morrison, Kim (2018) *The Art of Self Love*, Ocean Reeve Publishing, Gold Coast.

Morrison, Kim (2010) *Why Can't You Be Normal Like Me: An introduction to understanding the 4 personality types*. [eBook], Twenty.8, Queensland.

Müller, Melissa and Piechocki, Reinhard (2007) *A Garden of Eden in Hell*, Pan Books, Pan Macmillan, United Kingdom.

O'Meara, Cyndi (2007) *Changing Habits, Changing Lives*, 2nd edition, Penguin Group, Australia.

Pape, Scott (2017) *The Barefoot Investor*, John Wiley & Sons Australia, Milton, Queensland.

Perlmutter, David (2013) *Grain Brain: The Surprising Truth about Wheat, Carbs, and Sugar – Your Brain's Silent Killers*, Little, Brown and Company, Hachette Group, New York.

Pollan, Michael (2009) *Food Rules: An Eater's Manual*, Penguin Books, New York.

Pollan, Michael (2006) *The Omnivores Dilemma*, The Penguin Press, Penguin Group, New York.

Proctor, Bob (1997) *You Were Born Rich*, Life Success Productions.

Robbins, John (2007) *Healthy at 100*, Random House USA, New York.

Robbins, Tony (2014) *Money: Master the Game*, Simon & Schuster UK, United Kingdom.

Robinson, Ken (2009) *The Element*, Viking Penguin, Penguin Group (USA), New York.

Seligman, Martin (1995) *Learned Helplessness*, Oxford University Press, New York.

Stoessinger, Caroline (2012) *A Century of Wisdom: Lessons from the Life of Alice Herz-Sommer, the World's Oldest Living Holocaust Survivor*, Two Roads, Hodder & Stoughton, Hachette UK, London.

Tolle, Eckhart (2004) *The Power of Now*, New World Library, Novato, California; Namaste Publishing, Vancouver, British Columbia.

Ware, Bronnie (2012) *The Top 5 Regrets of the Dying*, Hay House.

Williamson, Marianne (2011) *A Return to Love: Reflections on the Principles of a Course in Miracles*, HarperCollins Publishers, New York.

Winfrey, Oprah (2014) *What I Know for Sure*, Flatiron Books, Macmillan, New York.

Wood, John (2006) *Leaving Microsoft To Change The World*. Pearson Education Ltd, Harlow, England.

Yousafzai, Malala and Christina Lamb (2013) *I Am Malala: The Girl Who Stood Up for Education and Was Shot by the Taliban*, Little, Brown and Company, New York.

CAST OF THE
EXCEPTIONALS

I encourage you to find out more about *The Exceptionals* feautured in this book. Many of them have been interviewed on *100 Not Out*. The *Exceptionals* are –

Albert Einstein
Alice Herz-Sommer
Andre Agassi
Angela Lansbury
Dalai Lama
David Attenborough
Dick Van Dyke
Florence Nightingale
Giannis Meli
Helen Keller
Hugh Jackman
Jack LaLanne
Jason Whitton
Joanna Meli

John Robbins
Leonardo da Vinci
Malala Yousafzai
Matthew McConaughey
Michelle Obama
Mother Teresa
Nelson Mandela
Norma Anderson
Oprah Winfrey
Paddy Jones
Paulo Coelho
Richard Branson
Rose Kennedy
Ruth Bader Ginsburg

Stephen Hawking
Temple Grandin
Turia Pitt
Victor Hugo
Viktor Frankl

Wang Deshun
Warren Buffett
Wim Hof
Wolfgang Amadeus Mozart
Yisrael Kristal

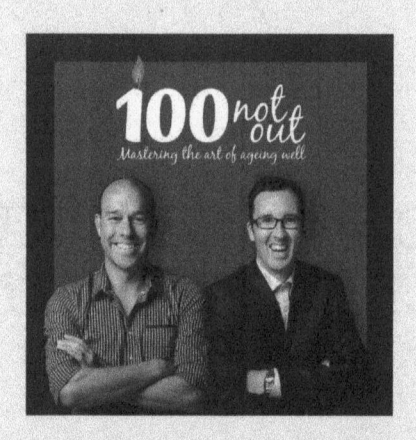

The Exceptionals featured on *100 Not Out*
(Episode number in brackets)

Ada Murkies (256)
Bill Stevens (220)
Bronnie Ware (39, 213)
Celina Biniaz (242, 243)
Charles Eugster (26, 115)
Cyndi O'Meara (40)
Damian Kristof
Dexter Kruger (17, 252)
Don Riddington (21, 22)
Eddie Jaku (103, 104, 244)
Heather Lee (30, 371)
Jan Smith (7, 84, 299)
John Demartini (3, 162, 264, 265)

Lavinia Petrie (28)
Kim Morrison (24, 405)
Madonna Buder (79, 82)
Marc Cohen (13)
Mimi Kirk (11)
Normie Rowe (268)
Ruth Frith (18)
Ruth Heidrich (27)
Sanduk Ruit (295, 296)
Thea Parikos (349, 372)
Thelma Zimmerman (317)
Tommy Hafey (2)
Trevor Hendy (61, 62)
Walter Bortz (5)

CREATE YOUR EXCEPTIONAL LIFE

12 WEEK ONLINE MENTORING PROGRAM

If you'd like the support of Marcus and a community of like-minded Exceptionals to create your exceptional life, this 12 week online mentoring program may be just what you're looking for.

Twice a year Marcus mentors a group of people to create their own Exceptional Life Blueprint. Week 1 and 12 is a 'Where Are You Now' workshop and weeks 2–10 focus on the eight areas outlined in *Your Exceptional Life*. This mentoring program is delivered online and can be accessed from anywhere in the world.

To find out more and register your interest for the next intake go to **marcuspearce.com.au**

BYRON BAY

Escape to the beautiful Byron Bay for a weekend of writing the script of *Your Exceptional Life*. Covering all eight areas of life, you'll create your own Exceptional Life Blueprint with the help of Marcus and a group of like-minded *Exceptionals*.

Find out more at **marcuspearce.com.au**

100 NOT OUT LONGEVITY EXPERIENCE

IKARIA
SARDINIA
BYRON BAY

Marcus and Dr Damian Kristof have been running the 100 Not Out Longevity Experience since 2016. What started off as a 10-day immersion on the Greek island of Ikaria has now expanded to the Italian Blue Zone of Sardinia and the Australian paradise of Byron Bay.

To find out more about upcoming Longevity Experiences go to **marcuspearce.com.au**

CONNECT WITH MARCUS

Book Marcus to speak at your next event

Bring the magic of *The Exceptionals* to life with a keynote presentation from Marcus. Topics include –

- The Island Where People Forget To Die: 10 lessons from the Greek Island Blue Zone of Ikaria
- Mediocre To Magnificent: 8 steps for personal & professional transformation
- The 100 Not Out Lifestyle: Wisdom from centenarians on how to reach triple figures (with vigour and spice)

For more information go to **marcuspearce.com.au**

100 Not Out podcast

Every Monday since 2013 Marcus and Dr Damian Kristof have been releasing an episode of *100 Not Out*. Whether they're interviewing a graceful ager or discussing a topic relevant to living an exceptional life, you can be guaranteed a laugh, a drop of wisdom and a great start to your week.

Subscribe and listen at **marcuspearce.com.au**

Your Exceptional Life Podcast

Each week Marcus discusses a key part of this book on his podcast *Your Exceptional Life*. Featuring re-released and updated interviews with *The Exceptionals* and the latest insights on living your exceptional life, Marcus discusses in more detail the principles outlined in the book.

Subscribe and listen at **marcuspearce.com.au**

Social media

Connect with fellow readers of the book in Facebook. Simply search for The Exceptionals.

Connect with Marcus on Facebook, Instagram and Twitter @marcusdpearce.

For media requests, bookings and all other enquiries, email **hello@marcuspearce.com.au**

There is more to the story in the INTERACTIVE book.

See exclusive behind-the-scenes videos, audios and photos.

DOWNLOAD it for free at deanpublishing.com/exceptional

ABOUT THE AUTHOR

Marcus Pearce is magnificently obsessed with helping people create their exceptional life.

A former smoking, binge-drinking journalist, radio and television producer, Marcus's media career included time at Leader newspapers, Sport 927 and SEN 1116 before concluding at Channel Nine and *The AFL Footy Show* in 2006.

Amongst writing hundreds of match reports, producing more than 1000 radio shows and dozens of *AFL Footy Shows* Marcus also covered major events including the 2004 Athens Olympics, 2006 Melbourne Commonwealth Games, the 2006 FIFA World Cup and multiple AFL Grand Finals.

His switch from sports media to health, wellness and personal growth media was seven years in the making.

In 2005 Marcus met his now-wife Sarah, a chiropractor, who was the catalyst of Marcus's health transformation from a Red Bull-guzzling, meat-eating smoker to a ginger-tea sipping teetotalling vegan, to somewhere back in the middle.

Marcus and Sarah spent most of 2006-07 overseas, living in a thatched cottage on 100 acres in Donegal, Ireland whilst running a chiropractic centre together.

On their return to Australia, Marcus and Sarah moved to Inverloch in Victoria to be closer to family, start a business, get married and have children. In 2008 they opened Pure Wisdom Chiropractic and Lifestyle, were married in 2009 and in 2010 and 2012 welcomed Maya and Darby to the world.

In 2013 Marcus and Damian Kristof began the podcast *100 Not Out: Mastering The Art of Ageing Well*. In that same year, Marcus joined The Wellness Couch podcast network as the Executive Producer of events including The Wellness Summit. Since its inception, *100 Not Out* has recorded more than 400 episodes and conversations with some of the planet's most graceful agers, high achievers and interesting people. *100 Not Out* has received almost one million downloads, whilst The Wellness Couch network surpassed 11 million listens in 2020.

In 2014 Marcus and his family moved to northern New South Wales. With Sarah now a stay-at-home mum, the time had arrived for Marcus to create the Exceptional Life Blueprint framework. He created an online program and began sharing his insights and trainings both digitally and in-person.

Since then, Marcus's online courses have been consumed by over 20,000 people in 155 countries and he has delivered keynote presentations and trainings to companies as big as NAB all the way down to local communities. Sectors including banking, health, wellness and real estate trust Marcus to help their teams perform to exceptional standards.

Not long after the birth of third child Tommy in 2016, Marcus and his podcast co-host Damian travelled to the Greek island of Ikaria – also known as 'the island where people forget to die' – to host the inaugural 100 Not Out Longevity Experience. Outside of pandemics, Marcus and Damian travel annually with a small group of people to experience the magic of Ikaria.

In 2019 Marcus and Sarah welcomed their fourth child Spencer, and amongst the craziness of raising young children, continue to love and support each other to make the rest of their life the best of their life.

ENDNOTES

Introduction

1. Levy, B. R., Slade, M. D., Kunkel, S. R., & Kasl, S. V. (2002) 'Longevity increased by positive self-perceptions of aging', *Journal of Personality and Social Psychology*, 83(2), 261–270. https://doi.org/10.1037/0022-3514.83.2.261

2. Ibid.

3. Buettner, D., & Skemp, S. (2016) 'Blue Zones: Lessons From the World's Longest Lived', *American journal of lifestyle medicine*, 10(5), 318–321. https://doi.org/10.1177/1559827616637066

Life Purpose

1. Ware, Bronnie. (2011) *The Top Five Regrets of the Dying: A Life Transformed by the Dearly Departing.* Hay House, Sydney, New South Wales. pp 37-47.

2. Kemp, Simon. (30 January 2020) 'Digital 2020: 3.8 billion people use social media', *We Are Social*, [blog] accessed 14 December 2020.

https://wearesocial.com/blog/2020/01/digital-2020-3-8-billion-people-use-social-media

3　Mohsin, Maryam. (6 August 2020) '10 social media statistics you need to know in 2020', Oberlo, [blog] accessed 14 December 2020. https://www.oberlo.com/blog/social-media-marketing-statistics

4　Ibid.

5　Galov, Nick. (21 November 2020) 'Social Media Marketing Statistics and Trends to Know in 2020', Review 42, [blog] accessed 14 December 2020. https://review42.com/social-media-marketing-statistics

6　Tromholt, M. (November 2016) 'The Facebook Experiment: Quitting Facebook Leads to Higher Levels of Well-Being', *Cyberpsychology, Behavior, and Social Networking*. https://doi.org/10.1089/cyber.2016.0259

7　Ibid.

8　Winfrey, Oprah. (10th August 2017) 'Paulo Coelho, Part 1: What If the Universe Conspired In Your Favor?' [podcast], *Oprah's SuperSoul Conversations*, accessed 12 February 2019.

9　Agassi, Andre. (2009) *Open: An Autobiography*, Harper Collins Publishers, London, p.28.

10　Ibid.

11　Clarke, M. (31 May 2013) *The Lady in Number 6*. Bunbury Films, Montreal.

12　Ibid.

13　Gripper, Ali. (2018) *The Barefoot Surgeon: The inspirational story of Dr Sanduk Ruit, the eye surgeon giving sight and hope to the world's poor*. Allen & Unwin, Crows Nest, New South Wales. pp 39-40.

14　Lehmann, A. C., Ericsson, K. A. (1997) 'Research on expert performance and deliberate practice: Implications for the education of amateur musicians and music students', *Psychomusicology: A Journal of Research in Music Cognition*. https://doi.org/10.1037/h0094068

15. World Health Organization. (2016) *World Health Statistics 2016: Monitoring health for the SDGs*. World Health Organization.

16. Tatlow, Didi Kirsten. (8 November 2016) 'Age Is a State of Mind for 'China's Hottest Grandpa'', *The New York Times*, p. 8.

17. Beautiful Music and Culture. (August 22 2016) 'Wang Deshun – Coolest Northeasterner (Inspirational Short Film).' YouTube video, 1:55, accessed 20 October 2019. https://www.youtube.com/watch?v=_IWtVDr6DCk

18. Williamson, Marianne. (1992) *A Return to Love: Reflections on the Principles of A Course In Miracles*. HarperCollins, New York. p. 165.

19. Farkas, S. & Johnson, J. (2002) 'Aggravating Circumstances: A Status Report on Rudeness in America'. ERIC, accessed February 19, 2021. https://eric.ed.gov/?id=ED463884

Movement

1. Shetty, Jay. (5 August 2019) 'Dan Buettner and Ben Leedle: On How To Design Your Life To Live Longer, Healthier and Happier' [podcast], *On Purpose with Jay Shetty*, accessed 21 March 2020.

2. Ibid.

3. Ibid.

4. Buettner, Dan. (2008) *The Blue Zones: 9 Lessons For Living Longer From The People Who've Lived The Longest*. National Geographic, Washington USA. p. 60.

5. Masters Athletics. (November 21 2009) 'Ruth Frith 100 Years Old In World Masters Games 2009', YouTube video, 1:44, accessed February 19, 2021. https://www.youtube.com/watch?v=FjkD21WxVEs

6. Ibid.

7. Ibid.

8   Buettner, Dan. (2008) *The Blue Zones: 9 Lessons For Living Longer From The People Who've Lived The Longest*. National Geographic, Washington USA. pp. 134, 275-279.

9   Ibid., pp. 275-279.

10 World Health Organization. (September 21 2020) 'Dementia', World Health Organization, accessed December 24 2020. https://www.who.int/news-room/fact-sheets/detail/dementia

11 Lambert, Catherine. (4 November 2012) 'Australia in danger of Alzheimer's epidemic', [Sunday Herald Sun], *Herald Sun*. https://www.heraldsun.com.au/news/victoria/australia-in-danger-of-alzheimers-epidemic-/news-story/9cf03a6bfcc4409829f78473122d8a6d

12 Xie, J., Brayne. C,, & Matthews, FE. (2008) 'Survival times in people with dementia: analysis from population based cohort study with 14-year follow-up', *British Medical Journal*. https://doi.org/10.1136/bmj.39433.616678.25

13 World Health Organization. (2016) *World Health Statistics 2016: Monitoring health for the SDGs*. World Health Organization.

14 Lim, J. K., Li, Q. X., He, Z., Vingrys, A. J., Wong, V. H., Currier, N., Mullen, J., Bui, B. V., & Nguyen, C. T. (2016) 'The Eye As a Biomarker for Alzheimer's Disease', *Frontiers in neuroscience*, 10, 536. https://doi.org/10.3389/fnins.2016.00536

15 Kivipelto, M., Ngandu, T., Fratiglioni, L., Viitanen, M., Kåreholt, I., Winblad, B., Helkala, EL., Tuomilehto, J., Soininen, H., Nissinen, A. (2005) 'Obesity and vascular risk factors at midlife and the risk of dementia and Alzheimer disease', *Archives of Neurology*. https://doi.org/10.1001/archneur.62.10.1556

16 Ibid.

17 Jeep Australia. (6 May 2011) 'Some 70yr Old's Don't Hold Back – Tommy Hafey for Jeep Australia', YouTube video. 1:00, accessed 4 May 2016. https://www.youtube.com/watch?v=M5OYIXIcbM0

18   Ibid.

19   Taylor, Denise. (2013) 'Physical activity is medicine for older adults', *Postgraduate Medical Journal*, 90, 26-32.

20   Maffetone, Phil. (16 April 2015) 'An Athlete's Impasse: Building Fitness Without Health', MAF website [blog] accessed 8 June 2019. https://philmaffetone.com/an-athlete-s-impasse

21   Kenrick, Chris. (10 December 2018) 'Longtime aging expert, now 88, heeds his own advice', *Palo Alto Online*, accessed 8 June 2019. https://www.paloaltoonline.com/news/2018/12/09/longtime-aging-expert-now-88-heeds-his-own-advice

Social Life

1   Berkman, L. F., & Syme, S. L. (1979) 'Social networks, host resistance, and mortality: a nine-year follow-up study of Alameda County residents', *American Journal of Epidemiology*, 109(2), 186–204. https://doi.org/10.1093/oxfordjournals.aje.a112674

2   Dalen, J. E., Alpert, J. S., Goldberg, R. J., & Weinstein, R. S. (2014). 'The epidemic of the 20th century: coronary heart disease', *The American Journal of Medicine*, 127(9), 807–812. https://doi.org/10.1016/j.amjmed.2014.04.015

3   U.S. Census of Population, 'Decennial Census of Housing and Population by Decade', United States Census Bureau; 1920, 1940, 1950, 1960, 1970, 1980, accessed February 2021. https://www.census.gov/programs-surveys/decennial-census/decade.html

4   Egolf, B., Lasker, J., Wolf, S., & Potvin, L. (1992) 'The Roseto effect: a 50-year comparison of mortality rates', *American journal of public health*, 82(8), 1089–1092. https://doi.org/10.2105/ajph.82.8.1089

5   Bruhn, John G. & Wolf, Stewart. (1979) *The Roseto Story: An anatomy of health*. 'Roseto in Historical Perspective', paragraph 4. University of Oklahoma Press.

6   Ibid., paragraph 16 & 17.

7   Ibid., paragraph 18.

8   Endo A. (2010) 'A historical perspective on the discovery of statins', *Proceedings of the Japan Academy. Series B, Physical and biological sciences*, *86*(5), 484–493. https://doi.org/10.2183/pjab.86.484

9   Stout, C., Marrow, J., Brandt, E. N., Jr, & Wolf, S. (8 June 1964) 'Unusually low incidence of death from myocardial infarction: Study of Italian American community in Pennsylavania', *The Journal of the American Medical Association*, *188*, 845–849. https://doi.org/10.1001/jama.1964.03060360005001

10   Bruhn, John G. & Wolf, Stewart, op.. cit., paragraph 1.

11   Maggio J (director) (2015) 'La Famiglia' [television program], *The Italian Americans* (Seasons 1, episode 1), Public Broadcasting Service, Virginia, USA.

12   Bruhn, John G. & Wolf, Stewart, op.. cit., paragraph 1.

13   Thomas, C. B., & Duszynski, K. R. (1974) 'Closeness to parents and the family constellation in a prospective study of five disease states: suicide, mental illness, malignant tumor, hypertension and coronary heart disease', *The Johns Hopkins medical journal*, 134(5), 251–270. https://pubmed.ncbi.nlm.nih.gov/4826123

14   Maggio J (director) (2015) 'La Famiglia' [television program], *The Italian Americans* (Seasons 1, episode 1), Public Broadcasting Service, Virginia, USA.

15   Ibid.

16   Hammond, E.C. and Horn, D. (1988) 'Smoking and death rates—report on forty-four months of follow-up of 187,783 men.' *CA: A Cancer Journal for Clinicians*, 38: 2858. https://doi.org/10.3322/canjclin.38.1.28

17   Friedmann, E., Katcher, A. H., Lynch, J. J., & Thomas, S. A. (1980) 'Animal companions and one-year survival of patients after discharge from a coronary care unit', *Public health reports (Washington, D.C. : 1974)*, *95*(4), 307–312. https://pubmed.ncbi.nlm.nih.gov/6999524

18   Hall, J. (2018) 'How many hours does it take to make a friend', *Journal of Social and Personal Relationships, 36(4)*. https://doi.org/10.1177%2F0265407518761225

19   Ibid.

20   Spiegel, D., Bloom, J. R., Kraemer, H. C., & Gottheil, E. (1989) 'Effect of psychosocial treatment on survival of patients with metastatic breast cancer', *Lancet* (London, England), 2(8668), 888–891. https://doi.org/10.1016/s0140-6736(89)91551-1

21   Ibid.

22   Miyagi, S., Iwama, N., Kawabata, T., & Hasegawa, K. (2003) 'Longevity and diet in Okinawa, Japan: the past, present and future', *Asia-Pacific journal of public health, 15 Suppl*, S3–S9. https://doi.org/10.1177/101053950301500S03

23   Loehken, Silvia. (2014) *Quiet Impact: How to be a successful introvert*, John Murray Learning, London UK. p. 7.

24   Galov, Nick. (21 November 2020) 'Social Media Marketing Statistics and Trends to Know in 2020', Review 42, [blog] accessed 14 December 2020. https://review42.com/social-media-marketing-statistics

Nutrition

1   World Health Organization. (2009) *Global health risks : mortality and burden of disease attributable to selected major risks*, World Health Organization. https://apps.who.int/iris/handle/10665/44203

2   Ibid.

3   Ibid.

4   World Health Organization. (1 April 2020) 'Obesity and Overweight', World Health Organization, accessed 28 December 2020. https://www.who.int/news-room/fact-sheets/detail/obesity-and-overweight

5   Singh, A. R., & Singh, S. A. (2008) 'Diseases of poverty and lifestyle, well-being and human development', *Mens sana monographs, 6*(1), 187–225. https://doi.org/10.4103/0973-1229.40567

6   World Health Organization. (9 December 2020) 'The top 10 causes of death', World Health Organization, accessed December 28 2020. https://www.who.int/news-room/fact-sheets/detail/the-top-10-causes-of-death

7   World Health Organization. (9 December 2020) 'The top 10 causes of death', World Health Organization, accessed December 28 2020. https://www.who.int/news-room/fact-sheets/detail/the-top-10-causes-of-death

8   Buettner, Dan. (2008) *The Blue Zones: 9 Lessons For Living Longer From The People Who've Lived The Longest.* National Geographic, Washington USA. p. 175.

9   OzHarvest (n.d.) 'Food Waste Facts', OzHarvest.org, accessed February 12 2020. https://www.ozharvest.org/what-we-do/environment-facts

10 Ibid.

11 Ibid.

12 Mitchell, H. H., Hamilton, T. S., Steggerda, F. R., Bean, H. W. (1945) 'The Chemical Composition Of The Adult Human Body And Its Bearing On The Biochemistry Of Growth', *Journali of Biological Chemistry 158*. https://www.jbc.org/content/158/3/625.short.

13 Kassraie, Aaron. (24 September 2020) 'USDA Warns Home Cooks About Dangers of Frozen Foods', AARP, accessed 1 October 2020. https://www.aarp.org/health/conditions-treatments/info-2020/cooking-frozen-food-safely.html

14 Cook, Jenny. (14 April 2016) 'UK adults eat almost 50% of meals alone', Net Doctor, accessed 14 May 2018. https://www.netdoctor.co.uk/healthy-living/news/a26375/uk-adults-eat-almost-50-of-meals-alone

Family

1. Hammond, E.C. and Horn, D. (1988) 'Smoking and death rates—report on forty-four months of follow-up of 187,783 men.' *CA: A Cancer Journal for Clinicians*, 38: 2858. https://doi.org/10.3322/canjclin.38.1.28

2. Russek, L. G., & Schwartz, G. E. (1997) 'Perceptions of parental caring predict health status in midlife: a 35-year follow-up of the Harvard Mastery of Stress Study', *Psychosomatic medicine*, 59(2), 144–149. https://doi.org/10.1097/00006842-199703000-00005

3. Ibid.

4. Ibid.

5. Ibid.

6. Ibid.

7. Ibid.

8. PrimeHealthNews. (7 December 2013) 'Alice Herz Sommer, Holocaust Survivor, Cancer Survivor – Inspiration to All!', YouTube video, 12:31, accessed February 2021. https://www.youtube.com/watch?v=DcNgEqTKvyk

9. Shady Abashy. (14 December 2012) 'The Power of Forgiveness – Gary Ridgway', YouTube video, 3:20, accessed February 19 2021. https://www.youtube.com/watch?v=f2_OOaP763k

10. Ibid.

11. Ibid.

12. Morrison, Kim. (2013) *Why Can't You Be Normal Like Me: An introduction to understanding the 4 Personality types*. Creative Wellbeing International, Mooloolaba QLD. pp. 7–14.

13. Ibid.

14. Chapman, Gary (2015) *The 5 Love Languages: How to Express Heartfelt Commitment to Your Mate*. Northfield Publishing, Chicago.

15 Gibran, Kahlil (1923) 'On Children', *The Prophet*, Alfred A. Knopf, New York, p. 21.

16 Institut National D'Études Démographique. (July 2018) 'Life expectancy in France', *Institut National D'Études Démographique*, accessed March 10 2020. https://www.ined.fr/en/everything_about_population/graphs-maps/interpreted-graphs/life-expectancy-france

17 Ibid.

Growth

1 Britain's Got Talent. (April 13 2014) 'Spectacular Salsa – Paddy & Nicko – Electric Ballroom | Britain's Got Talent 2014', YouTube video, 6:57, accessed February 17 2021. https://www.youtube.com/watch?v=hjHnWz3EyHs

2 Ibid.

3 Ibid.

4 Ibid.

5 Shetty, Jay. (3 February 2020) 'Jim Kwik: On How To Learn Faster, Remember More & Find Your Superpower' [podcast], *On Purpose with Jay Shetty*, accessed 10 March 2020.

6 Ibid.

7 Dobelli, Rolf. (13 April 2013) 'News is bad for you – and giving up reading it will make you happier', *The Guardian*, accessed 14 February, 2021. https://www.theguardian.com/media/2013/apr/12/news-is-bad-rolf-dobelli

Wealth

1 Australian Bureau of Statistics (23 August 2017). 'Microdata: Australian Census Longitudinal Dataset with Social Security and Related Information, experimental statistics, 2006-2011', accessed 4 February, 2021. https://www.abs.gov.au/AUSSTATS/abs@.nsf/Lookup/2085.0Main+Features12006-2011

ENDNOTES

2. Aged Care Guide (n.d.) 'What costs are involved in nursing homes', *Aged Cared Guide*, accessed 4 February 2021. https://www.agedcareguide.com.au/information/nursing-home-costs

3. Dunn, E., Norton, M. (2013) *Happy Money: The Science of Happier Spending*. Simon & Schuster, New York, pp 119.

4. Ibid.

5. The World Bank. (7 October 2020) 'Poverty', The World Bank, accessed December 29 2020. https://www.worldbank.org/en/topic/poverty/overview

6. Mahjouri, Shakiel. (7 November 2017) 'Oprah Winfrey discusses most difficult guests and life with partner Stedman Graham', *Global News*, accessed 4 February 2021. https://globalnews.ca/news/3847951/oprah-winfrey-discusses-most-difficult-guests-and-life-with-partner-stedman-graham

7. Whitton, Jason. (30 November 2020) 'John Wood on Changing The World' [podcast], *The Wealth Faculty with Jason Whitton*, accessed 21 April 2021

8. Ibid.

9. Sun, Leo. (18 November 2017) 'A Foolish Take: Here's how much debt the average U.S. household owes', USA Today, accessed 4 February 2020. https://www.usatoday.com/story/money/personalfinance/2017/11/18/a-foolish-take-heres-how-much-debt-the-average-us-household-owes/107651700

10. Finder. (18 December 2017) 'Australians' household debt nears highest worldwide', Finder, accessed February 17 2019. https://www.finder.com.au/australias-personal-debt-reported-as-highest-in-the-world

11. Clason, George S. (1926) *The Richest Man In Babylon*. Penguin Random House LLC (US) New York, p. 27.

12. Pape, Scott. (2017) *The Barefoot Investor: The Only Money Guide You'll Ever Need*. John Wiley & Sons, Milton, Queensland. pp. 66-67.

13 Ibid.

14 Clason, George S. (1926) *The Richest Man In Babylon*. Penguin Random House LLC (US) New York, p. 30.

15 Australian Bureau of Statistics (August 2017). 'Microdata: Australian Census Longitudinal Dataset with Social Security and Related Information, experimental statistics, 2006-2011', accessed 4 February 2021. https://www.abs.gov.au/AUSSTATS/abs@.nsf/Lookup/2085.0Main+Features12006-2011
Micallef, Cameron. (5 July 2019) 'Australians Super Ready: How many Australians are on the pension?', nestegg, accessed 17 August 2019. https://www.nestegg.com.au/retirement/planning/australians-super-ready

16 At the time of print the age pension in Australia is $944.30 per fortnight or $24, 551.80 per year. Relative poverty in any country is calculated by halving its median income. Australia's median income is $49,805. The relative poverty line in Australia equates to $24, 902. Therefore, Australians on the age pension (without any supplemental income) live in relative poverty.

17 Demartini, Dr John. (1989) *Prophecy I: Seven Inspiring Days Dedicated To Empowering The Seven Areas Of Your Life*. The Demartini Institute, Houston, Texas. p. 337. www.drdemartini.com

Spirit

1 Elisabeth Kübler Ross Foundation. (2020) '5 Stages of Grief®'. Elisabeth Kübler Ross Foundation, accessed March 27 2020. Used with permission — https://www.ekrfoundation.org

2 Smith, Ali. (2014) 'Unstoppable: Part one' [television program], *60 Minutes* (June 1, 2020), Channel 9, Sydney.

3 Frankl, Victor E. (1959) *Man's Search For Meaning*. Beacon Press, Boston, Massachusetts. pp 137–138

4 Ibid.

5   Ware, Bronnie. (2011) *The Top Five Regrets of the Dying: A Life Transformed by the Dearly Departing.* Hay House, Sydney, New South Wales. pp 37–47.

6   Ibid.

7   Mikulic, Matej (March 24 2021) 'Antidepressant consumption in selected countries 2019', Statista, accessed March 29 2021. https://www.statista.com/statistics/283072/antidepressant-consumption-in-selected-countries

8   The Business Research Company (April 17 2020) 'Global Antidepressants Market 2020 to 2030: COVID-19 Implications and Growth', accessed March 29 2021. https://www.researchandmarkets.com/reports/5017384/antidepressants-global-market-report-2020-30?utm_source=dynamic&utm_medium=GNOM&utm_code=mmlpx9&utm_campaign=1380453+-+Global+Antidepressants+Market+(2020+to+2030)+-+COVID-19+Implications+and+Growth&utm_exec=jamu273gnomd

9   Soto, A. M., Brisken, C., Schaeberle, C., & Sonnenschein, C. (2013) 'Does cancer start in the womb? altered mammary gland development and predisposition to breast cancer due to in utero exposure to endocrine disruptors', *Journal of mammary gland biology and neoplasia*, 18(2), 199–208. https://doi.org/10.1007/s10911-013-9293-5

10 World Health Organization (2013) *Global and regional estimates of violence against women: prevalence and health effects of intimate partner violence and non-partner sexual violence.* World Health Organization, accessed online 10 January 2019. https://apps.who.int/iris/bitstream/handle/10665/85239/9789241564625_eng.pdf?sequence=1

11 The World Bank. (17 October 2018) 'Nearly Half the World Lives on Less than $5.50 a Day', The World Bank, accessed February 1 2021. https://www.worldbank.org/en/news/press-release/2018/10/17/nearly-half-the-world-lives-on-less-than-550-a-day

12 The World Bank (7 October 2020) 'Poverty', The World Bank, accessed December 29 2020. https://www.worldbank.org/en/topic/

poverty/overview

13   Harris, Ben & Calder, Rosemary V. (28 November 2017) 'Low-income earners are more likely to die early from preventable diseases', *The Conversation*, accessed February 19 2021. https://theconversation.com/low-income-earners-are-more-likely-to-die-early-from-preventable-diseases-87676

14   Tolle, Eckhart. (2008) *A New Earth: Awakening to Your Life's Purpose*. Penguin Michael Joseph, England, p. 27.

15   Ibid.

16   Demartini, Dr John. (1988) *The Breakthrough Experience: A New Perspective And Paradigm For Life*. The Demartini Institute, Houston, Texas. p. 21. www.drdemartini.com

17   Ibid.

18   The Good Body (10 December 2018) 'Sleep Statistics Reveal The (Shocking) Cost To Health And Society', The Good Body [website], accessed 19 February 2021. https://www.thegoodbody.com/sleep-statistics

19   Roll, Rich. (12 June 2016) ''The Iceman' Wim Hof on why breath is life, cold is God and feeling is understanding' [podcast], *The Rich Roll Podcast*, accessed 24 March 2020.

20   Ibid.

21   ComRes Global. (14 January 2018) 'Tearfund – Prayer Survey', Savanta: ComRes Global, accessed December 4 2019. https://www.comresglobal.com/polls/tearfund-prayer-survey

22   Ibid.

23   Sherwood, Harriet. (18 January 2018) 'Non-believers turn to prayer in a crisis, poll finds', *The Guardian*, accessed 14 February 2020. https://www.theguardian.com/world/2018/jan/14/half-of-non-believers-pray-says-poll

24   Ibid.

25   Ibid.

PERMISSIONS

Special thanks to the following publishers, authors and individuals for permission to include copyrighted material in this book. All attempts to attribute and seek permission of copyrighted information have been made.

Excerpts from *The Top 5 Regrets of the Dying: Life Transformed by the Dearly Departing* by Bronnie Ware reprinted with permission from Hay House Australia.

Excerpts from *A Return To Love: Reflections on the Principles of A Course in Miracles* reproduced with permission of HarperCollins Publishers.

Excerpts from *The Barefoot Investor: The Only Money Guide You'll Ever Need* reproduced with permission of John Wiley and Sons Limited (Blackwell Publishers (Books) Limited) through PLSclear.

Excerpts from *Happy Money: The New Science of Smarter Spending* reproduced with permission of Oneworld Publications (London) through PLSclear.

Excerpts from *The Richest Man in Babylon* reproduced with permission from Penguin Random House LLC (US).

Exceptional Exercise 7.4 repurposed with permission from The Demartini Institute – https://www.drdemartini.com

The ABCDs of Negativity reproduced with permission from The Demartini Institute – https://www.drdemartini.com

Excerpts from *The Power of Now: A Guide to Spiritual Enlightenment* by Eckhart Tolle reproduced with permission from Namaste Publishing.

The 5 Stages of Grief® reproduced with permission from the Elisabeth Kübler Ross Foundation – https://www.ekrfoundation.org

Excerpts from *Rich Dad Poor Dad: What the Rich Teach Their Kids About Money That the Poor and Middle Class Do Not!* reproduced with permission from the Rich Dad® IP department – https://www.richdad.com

Image in 'Personality Power' used with permission (acknowledgement to Florence Littauer, adapted by Kim Morrison)

Excerpts from *The 5 Love Languages: The Secret to Love that Lasts* reproduced with permission from Moody Publishers.